# The A Word

*Living in Harmony
with my Alzheimer Risk*

# Irene Smith

**FP**

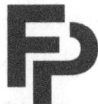

**Ferrishyn
Press**

This is a must-read book for anyone noticing any cognitive changes and wanting to take control of their own cognitive health. So many readers will identify with the author's initial dismissal of symptoms and I hope this spurs the reader into taking earlier action. This is such a moving story of one woman's sheer grit and determination to research and find her own solutions; one can only feel gratitude that she paved the way and is giving us the benefit of her learning across her health journey. As documented here, until recently there has been so little support for anyone wanting to take responsibility for their own health. We're sleepwalking into a health crisis, but this book gives so many tips for how to detox your world and live a healthier lifestyle, I'm sure it will help and encourage many people and not just those with cognitive symptoms, but with all manner of chronic conditions.

**Lindsey Byrne,** The Cognitive Health Coach

I loved this book— inspirational & empowering, the honest journey of the ups and downs of healing. There was a lot I resonated with, the challenges of wanting answers, the weight of responsibility we take on our shoulders when the medical system has a protocol that doesn't answer our questions, offer much-needed support, be able to provide an acceptable solution and at times dismisses our need to understand the root cause. With so much information on the internet, Irene, with medical training, navigates and explores the possibilities and shares her wisdom and findings of alternative and integrative ways to find healing.

**Jen Wilson,** The Healing Rebel

An important book with a groundbreaking message. Irene's book is a powerful story of courage and persistence as she takes us on her quest to uncover the 'why' of her illness and recover her health. And she doesn't pull any punches about what it has taken her to save herself from Alzheimer's. Irene brings together a great deal of information and research about the condition, its symptoms, and its cause and presents it in an articulate and thoughtful way. She ends the book with a rallying call for us to become more aware of the consequences of our current way of living on our children.

> **Fi Sutherland** Author, *Coming Home, Awakening Through The Stillness Into The Living Light*
> Teacher, The ISIS School of Holistic Health

Irene Smith is an exceptional health professional who implements the old axiom of "healer heal thyself". When faced with the all too familiar symptoms of Alzheimer disease, she knew, first hand, that the western medical model was of little help. Irene was looking for cure. This in itself is a huge leap of courage. The book takes you step by step through the twists and turns of setbacks and breakthroughs until actual recovery from all the symptoms associated with Alzheimer's disease. Irene's journey ended well and she gathered a treasure of practical information that shows there is so much more we can do to discover cause and therefore cure. The book is a huge source of inspiration that motivates the reader towards reclaiming cognitive health. It is incredibly well written, clear and easy to follow. As the number of dementia and Alzheimer's sufferers increases daily, this book is a ray of hope.

> **Fotoula Adrimi,** Teacher of Shamanism and the Path of Isis
> Best selling author of *The Golden Book Of Wisdom: Ancient Spirituality And Shamanism For Modern Times*
> Partner of The ISIS School of Holistic Health

Published in 2023 by Ferrishyn Press

ISBN Paperback: 978-1-7394386-0-9
Ebook: 978-1-7394386-1-6

A CIP catalogue copy of this book can be found in the British Library.

Published with the help of Indie Authors World
www.indieauthorsworld.com

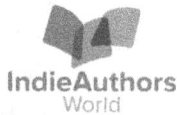

IndieAuthors
World

For My Grandchildren
and
In Memory of Jessie, Eddie and Nessie who walked this road before me
with no ReCODE.

# Acknowledgements and Thanks

This book began in 2015. Writing was constantly interrupted as life events took over and illness took me out of circulation. However, this was beneficial as on experiencing further cognitive issues, I found a route to recovery in 2019. That transformed the original writings into something more important.

I would like to express my thanks to a number of people. Thanks to the friends/clients who attended my Complimentary Therapy practice and suggested I should write about this experience. Without that seed being planted this book would not have been born.

To Indie Authors World who made the whole thing possible. Heartfelt thanks to Kim MacLeod of Indie Authors and editor Christine McPherson for their work on the book, understanding and support as health issues continued to interrupt progress.

Overall I extend my gratitude to any dentist, alternative therapy practitioner and conventional consultant who have helped me in any way back en route to wellbeing from 2013 till now.

My eternal gratitude goes to Dr Dale Bredesen and his research team for delivering their work to the world. Without the ReCODE Protocol I would never have made it back. Immense thanks to ReCODE 2.00 Health Coach Lindsey Byrne for your support and for guiding me out of the disorganisation I'd been living in these past years.

Gratitude to the unseen helpers in spirit who carried me through. I've been blessed beyond measure.

Thanks to my sons for putting up with me. You are the gift of this lifetime and I'm so lucky to share time with you, your wives and families. My love and thanks to my husband Ian. I was a tad fragile when we met. Thanks for hanging in there. And for the subsequent journeys we faced, I truly couldn't have done it without you.

# Introduction

This book began many years ago on the suggestion of friends who came to my complementary therapy practice, after I thought I had recovered from an episode of cognitive decline. Writing the book was a struggle, as my mother took ill around the same time as I developed cognitive symptoms, and my hands were full trying to help her. The symptoms I experienced were described on an Alzheimer's website as prodromal dementia, and there was no help available to me on seeing a doctor at this early stage. So I had to search for help myself, and I believed I had found a reason and, on improving, thought I had recovered. I was wrong.

The reality that I was wrong hit me when I experienced symptoms again in 2018. They came accompanied by an illness that floored me, making writing the last thing on my mind. I also feared I wouldn't overcome the cognitive problems a second time.

My paternal grandmother was the first to develop dementia. None of the family considered that more of us would experience dementia in the future, yet I was the fourth family member over three generations to experience symptoms. Medication hadn't worked for my relatives, so when it was clear that mainstream medicine couldn't help me either, it should not have come as a surprise. A journey that would last several years began.

At the time of writing, conventional medicine has no treatment to help reverse cognitive decline. My recovery is thanks to the integrated functional approach to medicine with help from mainstream medicine for other health reasons. Returning from cognitive decline opens the door to more possibilities for people experiencing diseases of these modern times. The more I learned, the more concerned I was for my children and grandchildren. I'm sharing my story of recovery as many people may not be aware the possibility of recovery exists.

However, I'm not in any way suggesting what people should do for their health. Nor am I taking a stance favouring conventional or alternative approaches to wellness, as I belong to both camps. I trained as a registered general nurse, and I've also leaned towards the natural approach to health. There is much to be gained from both areas of medicine, but I do believe we need a different approach and outlook for health than the one we currently have.

Many factors led to finding myself with cognitive decline, and I had to decide how much I would share in the book. The functional perspective uses the holism approach to medicine, considering the patient's timeline over a lifetime. It was not a straightforward decision to disclose private parts of my life. But such circumstances weaved the fabric of who I am, and I see some of them as steppingstones on my way to illness. My story, therefore, would be incomplete if I did not disclose some of this information.

In addition, my paternal grandfather embraced his intuition, and both I and relatives on that side of the family have had our own experiences. I believe we are all intuitive, but society's structure moves us away from our intuitive self, leading us to forget that intuition is part of our innate being. Others share my view. Razi Berry (https://naturalpath.net/) describes intuition as a part of our natural human senses but something we can lose connection with if caught up with the demands of modern living.

Intuitive sensing has accompanied me throughout life, and I never dismiss what I'm fortunate enough to receive. I've needed that innate part of my being, and it brought some insights on my journey of healing. Such experiences appear in my story because, like disclosing some private details of my life, this is also who I am. Anyone finding such accounts unrealistic, please disregard them. Healthy scepticism won't have any bearing on the experience I recount.

Alzheimer's disease has become one of the most feared illnesses of our time. The website alzheimer.org.uk explains that figures from the Office of National Statistics in 2018 showed the death rate from dementia has increased every year. In 2020, only COVID-19 moved dementia into being the second biggest killer in the UK since 2015.

Having witnessed dementia in several family members, I knew my symptoms were a concern since 2012 but received no treatment. When the problem recurred some years later, I found a medical approach that offered me a road out of cognitive decline. What if we can prevent Alzheimer's with the right education or appropriate medical intervention at the right time? This is my story.

Part One

# My Road To Cognitive Decline

# Chapter 1

# Family History

Gran Jessie was diagnosed with arteriosclerotic dementia, but Dad's diagnosis was Alzheimer's disease, which led to immediate early retirement for him at 63 years of age. Unfortunately, I can't describe his initial symptoms as my mother and I were estranged previous to this. I discussed the fallout with Dad before he became ill, and on learning both sides of the story, he told me to stand my ground. This wasn't unusual, as he'd often stood up and supported me when I was younger. Sadly, dementia followed, and by the time I saw him again, he struggled to make a coherent sentence.

I believe the way the whole situation unfolded wasn't intentional on Mum's part. She might not have recognised it either, or hoped it wasn't happening, rather than simply omitting to tell me. But I loved my father, and I couldn't have left him alone in his battle with this condition.

Younger than Gran had been, his deterioration into this dreadful disease was a quick, persistent withering, losing every faculty that made him Eddie. The consultant delivering the diagnosis told Mum that other relatives of Dad's might be affected. And indeed, his sister – my Aunt Nessie – was diagnosed aged 70, which I struggled to understand, as she had always exercised, smoked a little, ate a good diet, and was a healthy weight.

The difficulty of mending the bridge between my mother and me began when my husband, Ian, met my dad and brought him to my home to see me. A gentle person, Dad was close to his birth family and his children, and our reunion was poignant.

As he struggled to convey his feelings, he took a bottle of diazepam from his pocket – a medication prescribed for the anxiety he felt at the situation he found himself in. 'I'm going the same way as my mother,' he said clearly, and my heart broke for him. He was prescribed Aricept for his dementia symptoms, yet the deterioration was rapid.

Dementia care was still within the National Health Service in Scotland at that time, and Dad was in long-term care by the time he reached 66. He spent the next eight years of his life in a psychogeriatric ward, sitting in a reclining chair for his own safety. Aunt Nessie's deterioration was similar, but by that time care had moved to the private sector, so she spent her last months in a care home.

The pain of watching Dad's deterioration left me crying after every visit. When I learned that genetic testing for an associated gene was available, it horrified me and had me wondering who would want to know they might have such a future. My own efforts to keep well included stopping smoking in my late twenties, eating well, and exercising until health issues out of my control intervened, so I felt I didn't need to be tested.

Yet, in 2012, nine years after Dad had passed, I knew something was happening in my brain. By 2013, I had my first marked experience of cognitive symptoms. My long journey of seeking help began.

## My Life Before

I started nursing training in 1976, and began my secondment that winter in a medical ward. Back then, the wards were Nightingale-style, with beds lined up across from each other, and there was a short corridor before the ward opened into the patient area. On my first day on reaching the entrance to the ward, I stopped in my tracks. Ill people were looking across at each other, attached to nasogastric tubes, intravenous infusions, and heart monitors. I felt a sense of shock on seeing them, and was immediately struck by the thought that there had to be more to restoring health than this!

It was perhaps an innate knowing, but I never had that thought again while I completed nurse training. I staffed in the Orthopaedics department, dealing with emergency trauma and elective surgery, and it was the most enjoyable time in my career. Surgical and medical departments provided excellent medical care. Maternity departments took care of mums and babies. As I honoured and still respect the work within mainstream medicine, it never occurred to me that it is really an illness management system.

Patients are assisted in dealing with their situation, not necessarily assisted in restoring health. On experiencing cognitive symptoms, I thought back to that first day on a medical ward. There is still no corrective help available for dementia within conventional medicine at this time, and I was eventually to discover that my younger self had been correct. There is indeed much more to managing our wellbeing.

After our eldest son Simon was born, I took a break from working. Ian's job required him to travel by the time our youngest son Adam was born, and complementary therapies began as a hobby for me. When he was working in this country, Ian watched the kids while I took myself off on workshops.

An unknown medical situation was, however, unfolding in the background. I'd suffered gynaecological issues since puberty, but doctors advised that the pain I had developed would settle down when I had a family. The pain did eventually settle, but having a family didn't correct my hormonal plumbing. I had an ovarian cyst, mistakenly treated as irritable bowel. And greater pain took over as the cyst leaked through my abdomen and into the pelvic cavity. It became an extremely stressful situation.

I enjoyed the learning which the workshops delivered, and this took my mind off the worsening medical situation I found myself in. Remedial massage was a good fit for me, after working in orthopaedics, and I trained in the Bowen Technique. However, my heart lay more with energy healing, and I then studied Reiki healing. I became a Reiki Master in 2001 and had the pleasure of teaching Reiki to others, which I loved. I studied several other healing modalities, which benefitted me too, as a rollercoaster of emotion ran in the background of my life.

After the cyst was misdiagnosed, I had difficulty obtaining medical attention because of the confusing clinical picture. To manage the stress of this, I returned to nursing part-time. Once an ovarian cyst was detected, corrective surgeries followed, and I surprised myself in 2006 when, on a whim, I took on an office where I could work with remedial therapies. In 2010, hoping to expand my business by adding other healing modalities, I moved into a shop in a prime position in our town. Clients became friendly faces whose lives unfolded alongside mine over the following years.

## Chapter 2

# Emerging Symptoms

I n my early fifties, I noticed I was having dizzy spells. Initially, I didn't seek help because they were mild, but it wasn't lost on me that the same had happened to Dad. He had mentioned in his fifties that he was experiencing dizziness, but no cause was ever found. As his cholesterol level was high, he stopped smoking and started the low-fat diet recommended by mainstream medicine. Sadly, though, neither lifestyle change halted his decline into dementia.

My move to the shop premises was complete by September 2010. In hindsight, I now realise that signs of approaching cognitive decline were present, but I dismissed them. I never considered that would be my fate. To keep on top of things, I'd write myself reminder notes at bedtime, which then expanded into a notebook, and the following day I'd tick items off as I attended to them.

There was also a mild incident with money, which involved me giving my son the wrong change twice in a row for a purchase he had made for me. I paid close attention to ensure I did it right on the third attempt, and joked about such incidents, but I didn't laugh them off as senior moments. No, my catchphrase was "Oops Alzi Heimer", accompanied by a giggle. Little did I know that such symptoms signalled what lay ahead.

The most distressing symptom for me was misplacing keys, particularly as Ian could always find them even when I couldn't. He put this down to stress. Over the previous years, I had been called away from my family at short notice because of Mum's mismanagement of Dad's illness at home. She also caused other minor troubles with nursing staff once he was in care, and this all left me feeling exhausted and stressed. Dealing with these problems and witnessing Dad's decline meant there was a chance Ian was right, and the stress continued even after my dad passed away.

But the incidents with keys really troubled me. I did not seem to recognise the keys were actually there. The distress of this, believe it or not, led me to consider my house was haunted. Daft, I know, but denial is a huge thing.

There were no noticeable memory issues, and I continued to regard bedtime notes as something that kept me on track due to outside pressures in my life. As I wasn't too concerned about the dizziness, my intention was to seek help if anything occurred that I considered needed attention. I never for one moment considered I would deal with dementia symptoms in the near future.

An incident which I can only describe as neurological occurred on 29th June, 2011. Ian and I had gone out for a meal the evening before, to celebrate my birthday, but I didn't particularly enjoy the food.

The following morning, I fell over to the side as I was walking, and I initially thought I was suffering a stroke, but there were no other marked symptoms. I called Ian at work and asked him to check on me in one hour, then went back to bed. After a brief nap,

I appeared fine but felt I had sweats, and put this down to the meal from the evening before. The following weeks seemed to support this, as my gut felt upset and I could think of no other reason.

In 2012, during a second incident, I felt something whip across the left side of my brain while I was sitting in my kitchen. Shock forced me to my feet, and I flung myself across the beech kitchen table to avoid falling over. I knew this marked the start of something serious.

While I felt a doctor would not consider these symptoms a precursor to dementia, I still attended the GP to discuss them. As tinnitus was another symptom that had worsened over these years, she offered me treatment for Meniere's disease, which I declined because I felt there was more taking place.

About nine months after the whipping sensation in my head, I had obvious symptoms I couldn't ignore. I searched Alzheimer associations websites and found the symptoms I was experiencing were there, listed as prodromal dementia. They described prodromal dementia as the very early stage of dementia.

www.dictonary.com describes prodrome as: "An early symptom that signals the onset of an illness or disease; a symptom or series of symptoms that precedes the more obvious, diagnosable symptoms that develop along with the condition."

Memory problems joined my reminder notes and misplaced keys. One evening, it took me three hours to recall the name of a friend's niece. I felt anxious, irritable, or depressed, and wondered if it was due to the stress of previous years. Distress worsened on learning that losing keys or spectacles was a symptom recognised to almost always develop into an Alzheimer's diagnosis.

Things got worse when I started losing my way at work. On occasions, I would be working with a client when I was suddenly unable to remember the remedial moves I'd completed during the treatment moments before. Both at work and at home, I was forgetting tasks that needed my attention. I would sometimes struggle to remember where I'd parked my car at the supermarket, having to walk up and down the various lanes until I came across it.

In some respects, at this stage I still thought conventional medicine was the way forward. I returned to my doctor with my concerns, and bloods were checked for memory lapses, but they showed nothing significant. The search for information on causes of dementia was as I expected: healthy lifestyle choices regarding diet, exercise, and smoking. High blood pressure and stroke, and known risk factors for cardiovascular disease, are also risk factors for dementia. Cholesterol management, a healthy weight, low alcohol intake, and blood pressure control were the advice.

As these risk factors didn't apply to me at the time, I considered that something must have caused the cognitive symptoms, and I desperately wanted to discover what that something was. After my few visits to the doctor, it was obvious there was no help available for what I was experiencing. The enormity of this didn't register with me at first, but left to my own devices, I feared the symptoms may lead to dementia. So I attempted to find another way.

I tried to join research at the Glasgow Memory Clinic, who were looking for people with early signs of dementia and this would have given me access to tests, but they considered me too young. They offered details of other research I was eligible to join, but to my shock, that study would assess participants for ten years. And the entire research programme would span 20 years. This long-term research programme was no help for what was going on now. I knew I didn't have ten years to play with this situation, and additionally, removal from the study awaited if symptoms developed or if I received a diagnosis of dementia.

All research into dementia is, without a doubt, looking to help sufferers of the disease. But I questioned the value of research that took so long to return answers, if indeed it returned any at all. As the lack of medical help gradually sunk in, Google became a friend as I researched again and again for solutions to my symptoms. Years before, I had read a book about a man diagnosed with Alzheimer's disease who recovered after treating it as aluminium toxicity. I searched long and hard for this book but couldn't find it anywhere. All I found was a suggested link to mercury.

The realisation of no available help, and that removal from research rather than treatment awaited if I received a diagnosis, filtered into my reality. For some reason, though, I wasn't fearful at this stage, believing there must be a reason for my symptoms, as I didn't fit the mainstream view of predisposition. That spurred on my search, yet I could find nothing other than mercury toxicity.

Until that time, I had not voiced my concerns to Ian. But feeling I had maybe found an answer, I marched into the living room and announced that I thought I had mercury poisoning. Ian glanced up at me from watching TV as if I had a screw loose. I imagined a neon sign above his head flashing, "Aye okay, hen!"

Deflated that he didn't take me seriously, I returned to my laptop and decided I had to start somewhere. By 12.30am, my family were asleep. I poured myself a whisky and shed a silent tear for Dad and Aunt Nessie, who had walked along this path before me without hope of return.

# Chapter 3

# My Plight Begins

I n January 2013, a client who had attended my remedial practice mentioned his health had improved on removing mercury from his body. He had followed Andrew Cutler's advice, so I ordered Mr Cutler's publication. By now, I felt it was necessary to do something. While I found Andrew Cutler's book a great help, I skimmed through parts too quickly in my haste for answers to get rid of the symptoms. I found a practitioner who offered a Kilmer test – a challenge test that measures metals in the urine – and, of course, I did it as soon as I could.

Ian and I had booked a short break to Crieff Hydro, where we had been before. So I did the test on the Sunday morning before we left, and symptoms appeared by the Tuesday. That evening, on chatting with Ian about golf, I blurted out "golf sticks" instead of "golf clubs". The words felt as if they spilt out in desperation as I struggled to retrieve them.

We were having a drink in the lounge, and I left to go to the ladies' toilet. However, instead of reaching my destination, I arrived at a dead end. I'd gone in completely the wrong direction, despite having stayed at the hotel before. Disorientation to surroundings can be common even in the early stages of dementia, especially when in an unfamiliar environment.

On returning to the lounge, I smiled at Ian and acknowledged that I'd got lost. "I saw you go in the wrong direction, love," he told me. "What worries me is you didn't come back. Did you not know you had gone in the wrong direction?"

When I explained that I didn't think he realised how much this was worrying me, his response was, "I do now."

The following morning, I couldn't get out of bed. All my joints were painful, and I had severe brain fog and vertigo. I knew I must be reabsorbing whatever toxins the challenge test had moved. I later saw that Andrew Cutler advised never to do a challenge test, and by then I knew why. Judging by the severity of my symptoms, I had some type of toxic load.

Challenge tests, also called provoked tests, are used as a method of chelation. Chelation is a treatment aimed at removal of heavy metals if there is an accumulated load in the body leading to symptoms. There are arguments for and against its use and, from my experience, it's a treatment that a trained practitioner should oversee. In the test I did, I took a chelating agent as tablets which would increase removal of metals from my cells into my urine. The urine sample is then sent for testing to determine the amount of metals excreted.

One problem with chelation is that metal ions attach to the chelating agents which speed up their removal. If not carried out under supervision, this may be damaging to someone who has a heavy metal burden in their body. In addition, chelating agents can move more than metals alone.

I had contacted several practitioners for advice prior to doing the Kilmer test, but most were no longer offering chelation.

Unfortunately, I didn't know the reason why at that time, but found out later that our bodies have become so toxic that chelation itself was making people very ill. My experience made me realise that this process would be more difficult than I expected, as I struggled to find help.

A lady who'd experienced issues with mercury advised me to look for a holistic dentist for amalgam removal. This sounded a reasonable approach, as I had a lot of amalgam fillings, including in the roots of two crowned front teeth after a childhood injury. While I waited for an appointment, I tried anything I could find on the internet to aid heavy metal removal. But I felt so ill that a journal entry I made at that time compared my body to a folding bed that collapsed in on itself, which described exactly how I felt.

The dentist told me to stop everything I was doing. He, too, had stopped using chelation and explained that what I was doing was making me worse. Field Control Therapy (FCT) was the treatment offered. While there was some urgency to remove amalgam because of dementia symptoms, I was too unwell at that point to proceed. So FCT would start first.

The therapy determined that I had chronic mercury poisoning, as it was present in the bone marrow. Once I started treatment, an upset stomach and nausea improved, and the emotional rollercoaster I had found myself on eased. It made me wonder if previous feelings of anxiety could have been because of toxic influence.

Amalgam removal started a few months later, and I felt a marked improvement after 31 weeks. Anxiety when driving had gone, and brain fog had cleared. Misplacing keys also stopped around this time and, apart from a slight blip when I couldn't find a few things, that did not return.

As that was the one symptom linked to an eventual Alzheimer's diagnosis, I was so relieved. However, the blip was also a red flag. I would later discover that mercury toxicity was not the culprit.

# Chapter 4

# An Uphill Struggle

Alongside my experiencing dementia symptoms, my mum's health had started a slow, severe decline. It would be fair to say that she and I had never got on well, nor enjoyed a typical mother-daughter relationship. Apparently, I was the wrong sex, as she told me when I was 11 years old that mothers were closer to their sons. She also often reminded me that I looked like my dad's side of the family, which didn't suit her, so life at home was very strained throughout my childhood.

I invested time in healing from this with the help of my family and the many healing modalities in which I trained. And I believe this helped me to be there for her during her illness, because at one time I couldn't have managed this without it taking a toll on my own health.

Her various ailments, from minor health issues to kidney dysfunction and a cancer diagnosis, led to many hospital visits. And I could see my own symptoms were returning, but more mildly, with some brain fog and forgetting the odd thing here and there. The extra attention mum's illness gained her somehow increased her demands on everyone around her. She began starving herself – an unfortunate pattern I'd witnessed with her before – and she preferred a nightcap to help her sleep, so she didn't want pain medication. That's not a criticism. I might have made the same choice if I'd been dealing with her situation, but all in all it increased the stress I felt.

On returning from an errand for her, she would ask Ian or me to go for something else. Perhaps it was her way of letting neighbours see us coming and going, but the demands and excessive hospital visits were too much for one person to cope with, and it affected my availability to work and expand my business as I had hoped.

I thought that all this increased stress contributed to my symptoms, as I could not detox to the same extent. So I continued using various detox practices over another four years. What can I say? The world loves a trier!

In 2014 I found a practitioner specialising in treatment for heavy metals, but the programme set me back and culminated in my not remembering how to turn my computer on one day. I received no further advice after the treatment stopped, so I continued to try to help myself. But I was so involved with my mum's care that I didn't consider that perhaps I shouldn't still need to detox with amalgam removed.

Other methods I tried included advice on coffee enemas from a book on the Gerson Method, which the previous practitioner had started me on. I included salt baths, binders, contrast showers at different times to remove toxins, juice cleanses, and fasting, to clean my body further. But I struggled with fasting and had to abandon it. I also did Andrew Cutler's detox program, Hulda Clark's parasite cleanse – as I'd tested positive for a parasite with FCT – and Hulda Clark's heavy metal cleanse and a clay detox.

Every cleanse left me feeling unwell, except for Andrew Cutler's, but I had to stop it as a small amount of eyebrow hair fell out. I then tried detox Homoeopathy, which I felt helped my body to sweat. Toxic patients can have difficulty sweating due to the effect of toxicity on the autonomic nervous system. Its absence is a drawback, as sweating is an asset in detoxing. I was aware I had perspired little for years, but had always thought it was a bonus. How wrong can you be?

The homoeopath also felt there might be something other than heavy metals going on – perhaps a fungal situation or candida. My attempts at detoxing might have helped in some respect, but could also have proved harmful. However, I'd read so much about mercury staying in the cells, other metals binding to it, plus the difficulty in removing it, and I'd just carried on regardless.

I was in a state of desperation when I noticed symptoms returning and increasing in frequency. As well as brain fog with some forgetfulness, the bedtime notebook returned. One day, I parked my car in a temporary parking bay and, having opened up the shop, forgot to go back and move it. After work, I went to an adjacent car park and, of course, my car wasn't there.

On retracing my steps for that morning, I found it still parked in the bay, which I'd passed on the other side of the road on my way to the car park. It hadn't registered that my car was there! I joked with Ian about this, although he didn't find it funny and asked me why the symptoms were coming back. Poor Mum and her many demands got the blame.

I didn't seem to move forward work-wise either. I couldn't implement plans or build on the work I was doing, and customers often thought the shop was closed because I was attending to Mum's medical appointments. I was functioning in disorganised chaos but thought such unfulfilled plans had their origins in low self-esteem from childhood. When the shop's lease was due for payment one month, I realised I had come to a point where I could no longer manage if I was continually away from work for hospital visits. At the start of 2017, the fourth year of my mother's ill health, relatives helped with Mum's appointments.

I welcomed the reprieve, but I also felt incredibly sad. Despite our relationship, watching her decline was heartbreaking. She had been very active until succumbing to osteoporosis, although she pushed herself to go shopping until she could no longer manage. Breast cancer – found at the start of her illness – worsened, and needed surgery. Kidney disease, lung disease, an aortic aneurysm, and spontaneous spinal fractures, were among the other problems she dealt with. And she bore her lot with bravery, the memory of which stays with me.

My neglected home, with half painted doors and cluttered rooms, also yearned for my attention. The help I received with Mum's appointments gave me a little time to think about my self-care and the continuous detoxing.

Some things seemed to help, but at other times I experienced setbacks. I added clay baths to assist detox for a few months, but other symptoms appeared – abdominal pain, and fungal infection on my toenails. I considered I might have caused a candida overgrowth in my gut because of all the detoxes, so it was time to stop.

I also really wanted to get back on track with my work. Believing I had overcome cognitive symptoms, I was shocked when I noticed several errors in notes I'd recorded during the first episode. I had entered wrong dates on some, while other notes were only half completed. I did, however, still believe this was in the past.

In 2013, I had started recording symptoms in my journals, as I wanted a clear picture of which detox strategies worked and which didn't. On revisiting these journal entries, it was clear that my cognitive problems continued when I was back at work. In 2017, one entry read:

**31/1/17**

*Today is Tuesday. I can't remember what I made with two egg yolks on Sunday. I think the memory returned last night, but again today, I can't recall. Making muffins this morning, I would need to say I recall measuring a 1/4 teaspoon of salt and putting the salt back on the top shelf of my kitchen cabinet. Twenty minutes later when I go to get it, it's not there. But I put it there, and remember putting it there.*

*I don't panic, believing I'll come across it, like before. When I go back into the cupboard, it will be there, and I'll see it next time. Then I see the salt at the other end of the kitchen. Convinced I did not put it there, I smile to myself. There can only be one of two things happening. I either choose the reality that I must have put it there, and I can't remember, or, as I've considered before, there's some great big ghost taking the piss.*

*Two days ago, I tried a mayonnaise recipe (aha, two egg yolks) with coconut oil. This is the second time I've been able to remember this in twenty-four hours, although the memory is non-existent in between.*

I'd put these journal entries down to reabsorbing toxins from a cleanse I'd stopped four weeks before. However, I would later learn that my return to work was a significant factor.

My cleansing efforts continued to a lesser degree when I tried things like cleansing teas and barley grass, but barley grass and spirulina together worsened my symptoms. When setbacks included memory disturbance, I cut back on cleanses of any description. I dated journal entries for the beginning of February 2017 as 2013. And journal notes from March were noted as 2017 one day and 2016 the next.

As Mum's health declined at the end of 2017, there was no time for detoxing. I also realised that I was suffering from post-traumatic stress. It became clear there was no more medical help possible for Mum, so Ian and I needed to be around more, and carers were put in place. She had also refused to consider going into care, but this also changed.

When alone in the house, she imagined other people were there, which frightened her. End-of-life care at home was suggested but not put in place, as she did not want to be on her own at times. I would wait until she was settled at night before going home, then I'd go back down first thing in the morning. Admission to the hospital followed, and a room in a care home became available. But her deteriorating health meant she never made it to the care home, and she passed away in the hospital in April 2018.

## Clouds on the Horizon

Mum had certainly had narcissistic traits, and I recognised some characteristics in myself that could directly result from this – more so as I fell further into post-traumatic stress.

At the end of May 2018, I returned to work full-time. I stood in the main room of the shop and experienced what I can only describe as 'a blank', when I couldn't recall anything from a remedial treatment I had just completed. I blamed the stress I was trying to recover from, and I assessed other choices I was making in case I was doing too much. Information I'd found online about surviving the effects of narcissism led me to join a healing website, but I was growing extremely worried about myself.

Why was I continuing to have problems? Why did I feel I was recycling a toxic load? My clinical mind didn't enjoy being unable to join the dots, and attempts to quieten my thoughts were unsuccessful. Despite all my efforts over the past five years, I considered that I may indeed be on my way to Alzheimer's disease.

I was determined to return to meditation, as stress reduction had to be my priority now. Attempts to heal from what I considered to be the residual trauma from my relationship with Mum continued.

# Chapter 5

# Take Two

Symptoms persisted, and this time they had arrived unannounced. Problems with money followed. I'd bought goods amounting to £52. Counting out the payment, I counted £102. When the seller highlighted my error, I passed it off that I thought I had counted £10 notes rather than the £20s. I knew then this was an issue.

Fear centred around being unable to stop symptoms progressing and knowing there was no help available. It seemed that my previous efforts had achieved a delay but not prevention. In November 2018, I experienced the third neurological incident, which was much worse than before. I couldn't stand up straight when I tried to walk. My body leaned to the right and maintained that position throughout the day. It was time to share my concerns with Ian.

A painful tummy took me back to nutritional medicine. I went back to my GP due to cognitive issues, but blood tests continued to produce no answers. I still felt I had to inform my doctor. If symptoms persisted, I might run out of luck one day. If I didn't recover, at least I'd tried to get help.

I'd changed to a water filter, reduced plastic use, and my diet was 90% organic. Eco-friendly cosmetics and a reduction in perfume and hairspray use were added. Sometimes not knowing is worse, and my resolve broke a few times. I wondered if I had environmental illness because of insecticide exposure, as this had occurred previously. What was happening in my brain when I fell over and during sleep? It felt like there was no point in searching again. It was time to tell close friends I was having symptoms.

I had always thought I would never leave the church, even though my beliefs had differed from church doctrine. An incident, though, led me to decide it was time to honour them, and I found great comfort in doing things my way. I consider myself spiritual and sometimes wish I'd dared to step into my own beliefs earlier.

Using cards for guidance isn't a usual practice for me. But as I fell in and out of despair, overwhelmed as the reality of my symptoms hit home, I considered consulting Archangel Michael's cards. I offered a prayer for help, and the card I drew read: This is Your Life Purpose.

Many of us in the alternative therapy field may consider we have a purpose in this lifetime – not from spiritual ego, but from a genuine desire to help. My life has often been overwhelming, and I'd accepted I'd missed the boat for being of more service in the healing field. But here I was, with an Archangel I felt close to conveying a life purpose.

It was a purpose I didn't want, though. I had symptoms nobody wants. To have lived through often unfortunate experiences this time around, contemplating leaving it like THIS was too much to bear. I wept. As I cried, for some reason I thought of Jesus in Gethsemane, asking for the fate that awaited him to be taken away. I didn't have the grace to say, "Let God's will be done." I was too busy howling, "P-L-E-A-S-E... take it away."

The new nutritional practitioner I consulted asked me to forward any previous tests I'd had carried out. She explained that I had a previous B12 deficiency at a cellular level, rather than a blood serum level, and that this had a potential link to the neurological episodes. I'd also had a condition described as small intestine bacterial overgrowth (SIBO) four years before, but I hadn't been informed and it had worsened. The plan was if I could overcome the SIBO, diet would correct any B12 deficiency.

Some consolation came from the B12 discovery, yet I couldn't turn off a niggling thought at the back of my mind and started searching online. I came across information that functional medicine had considered a link between SIBO and Alzheimer's disease, so I initially felt hopeful that if I could overcome SIBO, my Alzheimer's risk might lessen.

Later reading highlighted that some research has suggested a relationship between various gut disorders and Parkinson's and Alzheimer disease, while other studies advised there was no confirmed link between SIBO and Alzheimer's disease.

Abdominal pain flared up intermittently from February 2019, which was widespread and felt inflammatory. I couldn't determine its significance, but previous experience with an ovarian cyst left me nervous to seek medical advice unless very necessary. I tried various things to keep the abdominal pain at bay, including starting the Gaps diet to heal the gut, and I focused on what to do about cognitive issues.

The weakness I felt made the diet a time-consuming and challenging transition, but Ian followed the diet with me for three months, which was a great help. I needed a great deal of support, and Ian cleared up everything and helped wherever he could, allowing me to concentrate on dietary requirements and cooking.

My mindset wasn't great, and I supported myself with Bach remedies. I started meditating with Insight Timer and continued with shamanic practice. My appointment with the nutritional practitioner was due in six weeks, and I didn't want stress to stand in my way. Despite my efforts to keep it at bay, abdominal pain continued and, on seeking advice from the nutritional practitioner, there was no response.

I purchased a webinar with a doctor who was an expert in SIBO, as I was desperate to help manage the symptoms. It highlighted the need to ensure my gut healed in full, but I couldn't settle. The potential link between the gut and dementia kept repeating in my mind. And I still couldn't believe that the episodes of falling to the side meant nothing to mainstream medicine.

## One Last Try

The sensations in my head led me to wonder if dementia patients experienced this but were unable to say. When the disease consumed my dad, I had initially been against genetic testing. But I'd come to realise that if I was heading towards Alzheimer's disease, it was time to face it. Ian and I discussed things, feeling genetic testing might be necessary, and he agreed we needed to know for our sons.

My feeling was that if I could get dementia, anybody could, because I'd really tried to look after myself. Deep down, I hoped I would find a solution. I desperately wanted to be wrong in thinking I was following in Dad's footsteps. Part of me still hoped I might get over this if I could manage the gut link.

Despite feeling scared, I searched again, not holding out much hope. But then it came – the possibility of recovery, based on the work of an American neurologist. The book was The End of Alzheimer's by Dr Dale Bredesen.

Hope, anticipation, and fear accompanied my buying the book. With no substantial treatment for dementia, I knew this book was my last chance. Medication had been of little use to my dad and my aunt, so if that was to be my only option, it wasn't a hopeful one.

After extensive research, Dr Bredesen and his colleagues had developed the ReCODE protocol, which the FDA (US Food and Drug Administration) rejected, and Dr Bredesen had taken his findings to functional medicine. I contacted practitioners he trained and who offered treatment for Alzheimer's patients and screening for anyone concerned about cognitive decline.

I wanted the screening, but by then I had become obsessed with genetic testing. I knew that many who carry the risk gene do not go on to develop Alzheimer's, and that some without the gene will, but I just couldn't get around the fact I'd experienced all of these symptoms again.

I contacted the functional medicine clinic to enquire about the screening in May 2019. My decision to initially delay the screening was because I felt genetic predisposition must be the reason I was experiencing this. If I didn't have the gene, it would be a surprise, knowing the symptoms I shared with relatives. I also didn't believe that all the sensations in my head meant nothing, and I wanted to be in control of my care if the day came that I deteriorated to that extent.

By that stage, I had been waging this fight for six years, and there was nowhere for me to go within mainstream medicine. But

I wanted my family to understand that prevention of Alzheimer's disease was a possibility.

The genetic results took longer than I expected, so I made my appointment for the screening, as I didn't want to delay any longer. It would be booked to take place on 12th August, 2019.

# Chapter 6

# The Screening

My cognitive tests showed a few areas with room for improvement, but nothing too serious. Genetic testing confirmed I had one copy of the APoE4 gene – a recognised risk factor in Alzheimer's disease. However, I decided not to worry my family at this point, until I learned more about the situation. I was advised the genetic testing also suggested that I shouldn't have a problem detoxing.

Results from an EEG and blood tests showed brain inflammation, the cause of which could be metabolic as abdominal pain had begun months earlier. I also had PTSD, which surprised me, as I thought I'd worked through it over the previous months. My endocrine system was making cortisol at the expense of other hormones, and the high cortisol also affected my blood sugar, which was higher than recommended. It was hoped these issues would correct once we sorted cortisol out.

The blood glucose level was just below prediabetic, which was the second time prediabetes had presented for me. It helped to know that cortisol was involved, as I didn't think it was due to diet. I had a vitamin D deficiency, which had also shown before. And a neurofeedback session confirmed age-related cognitive decline earlier than it should have presented. Finally, confirmation that something was taking place that wasn't just my imagination!

On considering the screening information, I felt I needed a brain scan. This would not be available to me through the National Health Service, because previous blood results for memory lapses had produced no answers and no referral was suggested. I asked my GP to refer me to a private clinic in Edinburgh to have a brain scan carried out, and this took place on 9th September, 2019.

I initially put off picking up the brain scan result from my GP surgery, but a telemedicine call scheduled to discuss blood results with the clinic changed that. On the morning of the call, I picked up the brain scan results, which confirmed damage in the white matter. It was reported as changes in keeping with what might be expected in this age group. But I had been eight years younger when this whole scenario started, including two neurological episodes in the first two years, so I was definitely not in this age group at that time. Despite my expectation, the shock of the result shook me.

I let the practitioners know on the Zoom call later that morning, and they reassured me I had caught this early and advised me not to get upset, as they could help me. Imagine the state I would have been in without such reassurance, having struggled to stave off symptoms for over six years. I felt very thankful and relieved by their support.

Ian and I booked a holiday for the following week, but I felt unwell. I appeared to be developing recurring sore throats and what seemed like an upper respiratory infection. Days before my holiday, I was working, and it felt as if my trachea was on fire. Abdominal pain became severe, and I tried to manage it with the SIBO information.

I emailed the scan result to the clinic, who got back to me quickly. The scan showed the start of paranasal sinus mucosal disease in the left atrium, which they told me suggested exposure to mould. We agreed that we could discuss this at my next appointment.

The sore throat and burning trachea went away overnight on leaving for holiday. As I relaxed in Spain, I had time to look into mould exposure online, and I discovered I had several symptoms. An intermittent smell had appeared in the foyer area of the shop, but I had been unable to detect its origin. I'd mentioned it in passing to the landlord, but it was never present when she visited. Years later, the smell became unbearable, and some mould appeared on the wall, but I had been oblivious to the dangers.

The landlord's handyman had eventually discovered a leak coming from an overhead gutter pipe outside the shop, and another leak rising from a drain on the pavement where the downpipe entered the drain. As a result, water was entering the shop. It took a few weeks to fix the problem, and a repair was made outside the building, but no work on the inside wall. The smell had gone, so I hadn't thought there was cause for concern.

On returning to work after my holiday, I felt unwell with a flu-type cold. Mould exposure became an obvious possibility by the time of my next appointment in late October. Abdominal pain was worsening, and I was distressed at feeling unwell again. In November, I felt worse as soon as I entered the shop, and had to cancel all work. I notified the landlord that I couldn't continue with the lease because of the mould. A decorative wall panel I had put up had proved to be a mistake, as mould had grown behind it due to the water damage.

On 18th November, one year since the last neurological incident, my test results confirmed mould exposure. One of the toxins in my body from the mould exposure could cause brain damage. This gave me a clearer insight into what had befallen me, and answered many questions.

My first visit for the screening had taken place three months before. They discovered the root cause in that short time, aided by the brain scan. Nursing training provided me with a great appreciation of what mainstream medicine achieves, but my education of a lifetime only began on experiencing cognitive decline. That's when my view of health, disease, and potential improvement or even recovery, underwent a complete turnaround.

Part Two

# The Return

# Chapter 7

# The Research

Research shows that several genes are involved in Alzheimer's dementia. However, the gene most recognised as raising the risk of developing Alzheimer's disease is APoE4. An allele is a gene variant, and APoE has at least three alleles: APoE2, APoE3, and APoE4. Features of the disease include amyloid plaques and neurofibrillary tangles, which prevent the normal transmission of nerve impulses across neurones.

Alzheimer's may have several contributing factors where genetics, environment, and lifestyle factors interplay. A carrier of the APoE4 gene will not automatically develop the disease, and people who do not carry the gene can still develop Alzheimer's dementia. And so a person may have no APoE4, or carry one copy of the gene from one parent or two copies, getting one from each parent.

The risk of developing Alzheimer's is 9% in people without the gene. This increases to 30% for carriers of one copy, and above 50% for carriers with two copies. The disease is described as late onset when developing in people over 65 years. This is the more common presentation, and there may not be a family history. Early onset describes the disease in people under 65 years, which occurs less often – in about 5% of people – and a family history is more common.

Amyloid plaques have been associated with Alzheimer's disease, and the theory has been that Alzheimer's is caused by amyloid plaques depositing in the brain. My understanding from the hypothesis I read back in 2015 was, to put it simply, that the supposition is that amyloid beta peptides cluster together and such clusters damage the brain cells. As the disease progresses, the clusters form plaques which are recognised as Alzheimer's dementia. However, the amyloid clusters themselves present a problem.

A synapse is a small area at the end of a neurone that allows the passing of signals from one nerve cell to the next. Neurotransmitters are chemical messengers needed to carry a signal across a synapse. While plaques are involved in nerve cell death, amyloid beta clusters ruin synapses before the plaques form. There have been changes in the hypothesis since I read that article, but the theory behind it remains much the same.

The amyloid hypothesis has been central to pharmaceutical research, but there has not yet been a drug developed that stops the disease progressing. Other research suggests that seeing the amyloid hypothesis as the causative factor of Alzheimer's may need to be reconsidered.

## Alternative Findings

In his book, The End of Alzheimer's, Dr Bredesen explains the process that occurs in Alzheimer's disease. He and his team of researchers found that amyloid is a protective response in the brain. Our innate immune system produces antimicrobial peptides as a first defence against infection. Other researchers discovered that amyloid also has an antimicrobial effect. From the point of view of protection, amyloid is what protects the brain from inflammatory threats. So, as long as there is inflammation, amyloid is going to continue in its protective role.

The plaques are problematic, but I learned from the work of Dr Bredesen and colleagues that the reason they are there has to be understood. Alzheimer's disease occurs because of factors threatening the brain. And if such threats continue to be repeated, the brain is constantly having to deal with them.

The brain then aims to safeguard itself with its protective response. The more the brain has to respond, the greater the risk of damage from its defensive strategy. To remove the plaques when threats remain means amyloid will continue in its role of protecting the brain in response to inflammation. Hence, the threats must be identified.

And the threats can be ongoing situations in our body that we are unaware of, such as a permeable gut, the presence of mycotoxins, and metabolic syndrome, to name a few – all of which I tested positive for. But it took nine years of mould exposure before I knew of their existence, and the early warning signs they gave me in 2012 of what was approaching, were not recognised by the medical profession.

Dr Bredesen and colleagues also found that Alzheimer's dementia is not just one undifferentiated disease. They initially recognised three subtypes in its presentation, and presenting symptoms differ depending on the subtype. Treatment, therefore, would depend on the patient's subtype. As research continued, another two subtypes were identified: type 4 vascular; type 5 traumatic.

# Chapter 8

# My Diagnosis

I do not have Alzheimer's disease; in fact, I have no diagnosis from primary care. The term applied there was memory lapses. Mild cognitive impairment was on the referral for the brain scan, and age-related cognitive decline showed earlier than it should have presented on a neurofeedback session. Brain scan results confirmed what I had been experiencing, and thankfully, ReCODE practitioners reassured me I had caught things in time.

The brain damage which I have due to mould exposure is white matter low attenuation (WMLA). The CT scan I requested, because of the screening findings, reported: "Patchy low attenuation change is present in the cerebral deep white matter and subcortical white matter." Not every Alzheimer's sufferer has WMLA, but CT scans have shown it on some patients with probable Alzheimer's dementia. It's been associated with severe dementia symptoms, and it's thought that Alzheimer's disease may have its own subtype of WMLA.

Factors considered to increase the risk of WMLA are high blood pressure, smoking, age, heart disease, and high cholesterol.

I stopped smoking in my late twenties and didn't have those other risk factors when my problems first started in 2012. The name for my health condition is mycotoxin illness, from exposure to mould in a water-damaged building. But it placed me on a path that could have progressed to one of the subtypes of Alzheimer's disease realised by Dr Bredesen and his team.

Tests confirmed I had Ochratoxin A and Mycophenolic Acid from exposure to Aspergillus and Penicillium mould. Ochratoxin A can cause adverse neurological effects and oxidative damage to the brain. It's toxic to the kidneys and the immune system, and is carcinogenic. I was advised it was this and not mercury that gave me the prodromal dementia symptoms I experienced, which correlates to the appearance of symptoms working in a water-damaged building. And it is a recognised potential factor in Alzheimer's and Parkinson's disease.

I was unsure if I would need to get rid of my equipment in the shop due to the mould, so I sought advice from a specialist company. The guy who came out told me I was overthinking the association between mould exposure and dementia. But he couldn't stop coughing, while stressing that it had nothing to do with the mould he was standing in front of. Time will tell.

With all the information I had gathered from test results, I knew I wasn't overthinking. And in the words of Dr Bredesen, "Alzheimer's disease due to mould? Sadly, there is more and more evidence that moulds contribute to some cases, likely at least 500,000 cases in the United States alone."

I needed a medical approach that understood such things, that could guide me from this point: removing exposure; strengthening my body to help me heal; overseeing safe toxin removal; and advice on the optimal diet to aid my recovery. Mainstream medicine doesn't work like that.

I now know why I'd felt as if I was recycling toxins, and can better understand the disorganisation, distraction, and low self-esteem. The one condition I'd never considered myself at risk from had come knocking on my door and turned my understanding of health and disease on its head.

As a carrier of the APoE4, however, it would be folly to think that mould was my only risk factor. I now know the other threats that could cause Alzheimer's disease to affect me, and naturally I want to ensure that doesn't happen. Only functional integrative medicine, also known as precision medicine, can offer me a way to fend off symptoms of Alzheimer's disease based on my individual risk.

## Interpreting my Screening Results

The screening highlighted factors that may affect my brain health. They include gut issues, low vitamin D, gluten sensitivity, prediabetes, cholesterol issues, and cortisol/PTSD. I feel, given the number of factors discovered, that I would probably have developed dementia at some point. The initial three subtypes discovered by Dr Bredesen and colleagues are detailed in The End of Alzheimer's book. In layperson's terms, I'll explain how the factors discovered in the screening relate to the possibility of my succumbing to any of them. Those subtypes are:

**Type 1** – inflammatory. In addition, there is a type 1.5
**Type 11** – atrophic
**Type 111** – toxic

Type 1 involves inflammation, which may come from food – the processed diet in particular. Other inflammatory agents include microbes, viruses, bacteria, and tick-borne infections or sources of inflammation in the body, poor oral health being one example. It usually presents with memory problems.

An EEG showed inflammation was present in my brain. I had developed abdominal pain which felt inflammatory, so this was a possible factor, and the toxins from mould can also start an inflammatory process which may affect the nervous system. Mould exposure can also lead to spores colonising in the sinus and gut, leading to infection. However, I couldn't tell if this had happened in my gut at that time. Inflammation can predispose me to inflammatory subtype 1.

Trophic factors help maintain and regulate organ function. Some factors supporting brain health include vitamins D and B12, hormones, and nutrients, and their absence affects the normal working of brain synapses. In type 11, atrophic, such support isn't available for various reasons. Its presentation also usually involves memory issues.

I was advised high cortisol levels were affecting other hormones, and a lack of hormones and vitamin D deficiency become atrophic factors for me. Some surgical procedures also affect vitamin D assimilation, and I had a hysterectomy, which is one of them. These contributors lay the foundation for subtype 11.

Type 1.5 combines factors from both type 1 and type 11. It's sugar-related, and prediabetes may be present, leading to insulin resistance. Sugar contributes to the inflammatory factor of type 1, with the insulin resistance belonging to the atrophic type 11. I showed a tendency to prediabetes, which emerged for the first time in 2014 when I was struggling to get help with cognitive issues myself. If this had continued, it could have led to inflammatory plus atrophic factors as described in subtype 1.5.

The subtype I was in danger of developing was type 111 toxic Alzheimer's. Type 111 involves exposure to toxins and affects executive function skills. Executive function skills help us with social interaction, planning and focusing on tasks, organisational skills, time management, etc. People succumbing to type 111 are more compromised than the other subtypes, as these skills are necessary for navigating our daily lives.

They may have difficulty in retrieving words, and visual perception can be affected. Memory issues, though, are not always a symptom of this type, and it can also present in a younger age group. In Alzheimer's disease, brain scans show downsizing associated with the disease process. In the toxic subtype, brain scans show indiscriminate damage, confirming exposure to some form of toxic agent. Mould excretes mycotoxins which can be harmful to health. I was surprised to learn toxic Alzheimer's occurs more in people with no family history of the disease, but should there be a family history, the person will carry the APoE4 gene.

Having discovered I carry one copy of the APoE4, I already knew it was risk factor for Alzheimer's disease. I learned the APoE2 and APoE4 may also contribute to heart disease, which certainly matches the family history on my dad's side of the family. Through a SelfDecode APoE DNA Wellness Report, I discovered the APoE protein is involved with fat metabolism and transport. My cholesterol levels were considered to be on the high side and would need to be reviewed, as cholesterol levels can pose a risk for dementia. Other predisposing factors need a little more in-depth explanation.

# Chapter 9

# My Other Contributors

P hysiology studies how the body works and how some systems and organs interact with each other. Our central nervous system (CNS) comprises the spinal cord and the brain. The enteric nervous system (ENS) is within the gastrointestinal system. There is a two-way link between these two systems, called the gut-brain axis, and the resulting two-way communication allows them to influence each other.

Our gut flora is an organ in its own right, and its combined genetic material is called the microbiome. Gut flora also has a role in communication between the ENS and CNS, and this interaction between the gut microbiota and the brain occurs through the gut-brain axis. There is also interaction through the vascular system, allowing access through the blood-brain barrier.

The gut-brain connection led to the consideration that Alzheimer's disease may also link to intestinal dysbiosis. It's known that inflammation can be a factor in Alzheimer's disease, and dysbiosis of the gut flora can lead to systemic inflammation.

Gut microbiota can cause brain dysfunction, and so an imbalance in the gut flora may be one predisposing factor. As previously mentioned, research has advised no established link between SIBO and Alzheimer's disease. However, SIBO is a form of dysbiosis, and tests confirmed I had SIBO.

Our gut flora is also essential to our wellbeing – being involved in digestion, manufacturing vitamins and nutrients – and the immune system. When we're exposed to pathogens, gut flora helps to defend us. In addition, probiotics are available through an appropriate diet, while poor diet, stress, and antibiotic use can make the gut flora less efficient. As well as Alzheimer's dementia, studies have shown that altered gut flora may be involved with degenerative neurological conditions, such as Huntington's disease, Parkinson's, and Multiple Sclerosis. All very serious outcomes.

## Leaky Gut

Leaky gut is a shorter term for gastrointestinal permeability, which functional testing confirmed I had. The gut wall is the barrier between you and your bloodstream, providing a defence against toxins and microbes getting into your system. Lipopolysaccharides are such toxins that can be detrimental to health if they pass through a leaky gut. They are a major contributor to low grade inflammation in the body.

The cells of the intestines are close together and, assisted by essential proteins, form tight junctions. In gut permeability, the junctions separate, allowing food particles and bacteria to get through. Cytokines are like an alert system signalling immune cells to fight such particles and bacteria.

If inflammation is present, it can affect the microvilli of the gut lining, compromising their function in digestion and absorption, and contribute to a leaky gut. Other factors that may lead to leaky gut include food sensitivities, infections including SIBO, poor diet, stress, medications, and low stomach acid. Low stomach acid can increase the chance of infections, highlighting that antacids and proton pump inhibitors may be putting our gut health at risk.

The role of the blood-brain barrier is protection from toxins and infectious agents that could cause disease, while allowing in nutrients and maintaining balanced conditions within the brain. Just as the gut has its defensive gut wall, the blood-brain barrier also has tight junctions. While this barrier is aided in its protective function in what it lets through, if leaky gut occurs, this can lead to a leaky blood-brain barrier.

## The Gluten Issue

Foods that are linked with food intolerance include grains, wheat, nuts, dairy, and eggs. The cause of food intolerance isn't definite, but one thought is that as our food has changed so much, the body doesn't recognise it as a food source. The body sees modern food additives as foreigners and responds by making antibodies to such additives and the foods that contain them.

Mainstream medicine can diagnose coeliac disease – a genetic disease with an allergic reaction to gluten. However, conventional practitioners may not recognise non-coeliac gluten sensitivity, and some may even dismiss it as a ruse. Yet it's becoming very common, with many associated health problems.

There are two proteins in gluten – gluten and gliadin – with gliadin contributing to a whopping 70% of the gluten protein. Antibodies in reaction to gliadin can cause reactions in the body that damage the brain and are associated with neurological conditions. Non-coeliac gluten sensitivity can also be involved in autoimmune conditions. My blood tests showed sensitivity to the gliadin protein.

Coeliac disease can damage the lining of the intestines, while gliadin sensitivity may not. However, it can give rise to symptoms mistaken for irritable bowel, and gut permeability may occur. There can be sensitivity to any of the 12 components within the gliadin protein. Dr David Perlmutter has an image of an MRI of the brain in his book, Grain Brain. It shows the same white matter damage from gluten sensitivity that I've sustained due to Ochratoxin A. So I need to consider that a lifetime exposure to gliadin might well have played a role in developing cognitive issues at a later age for me.

The conventional approach may suggest dietary measures to determine if a sensitivity exists. Improvement in symptoms with gluten removal, and the return of symptoms on reintroducing gluten, may suggest non-coeliac gluten sensitivity. Functional medicine can test for gluten sensitivity. Doctors Data and Cyrex Labs do detailed testing, and the test can be done through a functional medicine practitioner.

It doesn't always follow that people with gliadin sensitivity will be sensitive to gluten. But the removal of the gliadin protein alone isn't possible, so avoiding gluten is the only way to manage it. Genetics may also play a part in susceptibility, especially in people of Northern European descent, and my paternal grandmother was from Lithuania. I later discovered gluten intolerance is commonplace in people with Scottish, English, or Irish ancestry. So, a double whammy, as my mother told me her ancestors came from Ireland.

Due to the damage gliadin has the potential to cause, I wasn't reluctant to go gluten free. I found the initial transition the difficult part, and there's support online from people already benefiting from gluten removal. Not all gluten-free products are a great way forward for me, as many of them are still a refined starch, and I need to consider blood sugar levels.

## Cortisol

The screening showed that I still had post-traumatic stress. It's thought that stress has some part in developing dementia, but as it is a part of modern living, it's something we are all exposed to. When confronted with a stressor, the body signals the fight-or-flight response. During this response, the release of cortisol takes place.

Blood sugar levels increase on the release of cortisol, and cortisol is involved in how the brain uses glucose to manage stress. Most of the time, the flight or fight reaction is a response which the body resolves itself. On the stressor subsiding, cortisol levels reduce and the body regains equilibrium. However, with exposure to repeated stressors, there is no resolution. This disrupts many body functions, including the brain, and can lead to cognitive impairment.

Stress can affect the brain in many ways. A weakened blood-brain barrier can occur, which allows inflammatory proteins to access the brain. Shrinkage in the prefrontal cortex may happen, which is an area involving learning and memory. And the hippocampus, which is affected by Alzheimer's disease, can shrink. It's also known that stress can enlarge an area of the brain called the amygdala, making the brain more susceptible to stress, leading to a constant stress response. The effect of cortisol on synapses can lead to withdrawing from social interaction.

Stress can also affect other body structures, such as the cardiovascular, reproductive, and digestive systems. A high amount of stress or prolonged stress can be a factor in dysbiosis in the gut, and the effect on the immune system can make us more liable to infection. High cortisol levels have also been linked to disturbed sleep and weight gain, and adequate sleep is necessary for brain health.

# Chapter 10

# The Way Back

The ReCODE protocol stands for reversing cognitive decline. It has helped people to reverse cognitive issues and to maintain the benefits gained. Assessment of all the markers considered to be involved in cognitive decline takes place in the screening, allowing recognition of individual predisposing factors.

The contributing factors from the subtypes may differ from person to person. The interaction between genetics and the environment will also be specific to an individual, ensuring the protocol is tailor-made to those findings. As explained in the presence of unidentified inflammatory threats, amyloid will continue to form, and identification of the subtypes leads to a greater understanding of predisposing factors.

I started a vitamin D supplement and had some neurofeedback for PTSD. I was progressing on the Gaps diet and continued to read for advice on healing my gut. A SIBO compliant probiotic was begun and herbal medicine tailored to my symptoms. Once tests confirmed the root cause of cognitive issues to be mould exposure, I also started treatment for mycotoxin illness. I recommenced detox methods I was familiar with and got a portable infrared sauna for use at home. However, the infrared sauna seemed to mobilise too many toxins at that point.

I developed a tightness in my chest because of the mould, which I felt was similar to a mild asthmatic reaction. My doctor arranged a referral for a spirometry test which measures lung function. I hoped the abdominal pain that had appeared would settle on dealing with the mycotoxins. Tests later showed candida and a fungal infection in the gut.

As the months progressed, I felt improvement, although I couldn't explain in what way. I tried to return to work in different premises in February 2020, then Covid struck, and the shop closed for a time from March that year. While lockdown curtailed my return to work, it provided me with the opportunity to attend to getting back on my feet. I suppose it's strange that it had to take a lockdown to give myself the care I needed, but it did. If I wanted to recover, I needed to consider this.

Despite yoga practice, the improvement in my flexibility was minimal, so I felt the toxins might be in my muscles. Exercise seemed to aggravate abdominal discomfort, but it was mild and the only way forward. But by May, the muscle pain eased. My diet had moved on from the initial stage of the Gaps diet, and everything felt positive. I still felt shock that I'd actually been attempting to stem off dementia, and I needed some time to come to terms with my feelings around that.

Lists were no longer needed as much by the end of May, but it surprised me to realise that I had withdrawn socially. The brain map results from the initial screening showed there might be a reduction in social interaction, but I hadn't noticed it. There was an improvement in my cognition, though, and I had a definite sense I was emerging from something. Some months later, on tolerating infrared saunas, I could see I had further mental clarity. This surprised me a little, because by that point I thought I was fine, but it was clear there was further lucidity.

I closed the shop in July 2020, as the building did not meet Covid guidelines, and that allowed me to concentrate more on my health. In the months since the discovery of mycotoxins, dizziness and joint pain had settled and fatigue had eased. Abdominal pain had improved, and digestive issues and head pains were lessening. I could now focus and get things done.

My grandsons came to stay one night in September, and it was wonderful to interact and play with them. The experience was so far removed from Boxing Day 2016, when I had lain on the couch feeling so unwell from continued detoxing that I was ready to give up. At that time, Alfie had turned six, and Leo would arrive the following March. On that particular day, I was sick of my struggle, and the uncertainty of what the future held didn't bear thinking about. Then I thought of Alfie and baby Leo, who was on his way. The idea of being unable to interact with them, perhaps even recognise them, gave me the impetus to try again.

Now, though, I was getting some of my life back, and there was some time for meditation and spiritual reading. But suddenly one day, a low mood descended out of nowhere. Bach remedies helped me balance my mood until what I'm going to call crazy thoughts interrupted my peace. I'd previously related such thoughts to dealing with my mum's situation, but now I wondered if they were linked to mycotoxins.

My next clinic appointment confirmed this, allowing the practitioners to help me with it. People with environmental illnesses often find their symptoms unrecognised, so such support was really helpful.

Covid delayed the referral for a spirometry test, so I decided to try the Wim Hof breathing method for the tightness I sometimes felt in my chest, to see if I could gain any improvement. It helped, and a slight cough replaced the constriction. Once a date for the spirometry test was available, the difference in my breathing before and after a dose of Ventolin was minute. The test was, therefore, reported as normal, and I felt I'd passed another hurdle.

Setbacks, though, are tough to work through. Having enjoyed some improvement, I felt my energy failing by the end of September 2020. In addition, it was almost as if doing the Wim Hof breathing had caused my body to request more oxygenation. My cells were shouting out for me to walk and aid this, so I downloaded a walk for fitness programme from Jog Scotland. I introduced myself to power walking over ten weeks, and initially spinal and muscle pain eased.

However, familiar symptoms reappeared, and as I didn't understand why, I didn't deal with them well. My ears leaked a little, hissing in my ears increased, and I was experiencing a level of deafness. In the following weeks, fatigue joined in and muscle aches returned. I went back to the drawing board regarding my detox strategies, but I didn't think to contact the practitioners for advice.

The more I walked, the weaker I felt. Stiffness ceased to be relieved by stretching. Heavy legs, accompanied by severe joint pain, returned and disturbed my sleep. My throat felt like cut glass, and symptoms of a cold appeared, which I considered could be a healing crisis. I used all the detox strategies I knew and considered stopping walking, but continued as on another level I enjoyed being able to do it.

Dizziness interrupted my days. There was occasional insomnia, and my ears leaked to the point that I knew probably indicated I'd mobilised too many toxins. I just hoped the accompanying deafness wasn't permanent. Joint pain remained. I'd had previous experience of deafness some days while exercising to DVDs at home, but didn't recognise the significance.

Week ten coincided with my next clinic appointment, and I was told to stop walking immediately.

The onset of ear problems led to an audiology appointment, antibiotics from my doctor, and an ENT referral. ENT appointments were ongoing. No immediate improvement came from my enthusiasm to get oxygen into my cells, but what I learned from this would bring its own benefits.

I'd been advised that initial results received from genetic testing indicated I should have been able to detox without difficulty, but the practitioners looked again at the genetic results to see if they could help me further. Genetic testing gives information on genetic potential, but the gene may not be activated. Genes can be turned on or off for various reasons, and the term used when turned on is that the gene is being expressed.

Even if there is a risk associated with a genotype which a person carries, it is not a given that they will develop that health condition. Other factors, such as environmental influences and lifestyle, will contribute to health issues developing.

As explained earlier, an allele is a gene variant, and I discovered an SNP (snip) can be present in an allele. SNP stands for single nucleotide polymorphism, the term for when there is an anomaly in genes. I was found to have an SNP on the MTHFR gene. Having an SNP doesn't mean the gene doesn't work, but this mutation meant my ability to detox had the potential to reduce by as much as 40% if my diet was low in folate. This was not good after being exposed to mould.

As I didn't seem to bounce back from the effects that walking produced, I reassessed my detox plan and added cold showers, because they help support the lymphatics, and to remove candida from the body. Gentle stretching and walking were all I could do, and I only managed a short sauna of 7-10 minutes each week. Ian helped me at home as much as he could as, on some level, I felt myself slip back. I didn't seem to have any energy, and I knew I could not push my body to do more.

As Covid restrictions lifted, it was time to get lab work repeated in July 2021. It was also time to get the advice of a nutritionist to see if anything else could be holding me back. The lab work highlighted dehydration, which I found unbelievable because I paid close attention to my water intake. However, in my efforts to restore my health, I had learned to drink green tea for its reported benefits. But I now discovered that its overconsumption could be dehydrating. On top of this, I was deficient in magnesium, and I was leaning towards anaemia. Despite my best efforts, my LDL cholesterol was still above the recommended level.

Dietary adjustments which I made to support the SNP on the MTHFR gene seemed to help. I corrected the dehydration, and I built up gentle walks. At the end of November, I was walking four times a week with no adverse symptoms. I ditched enemas but continued with cold showers and saunas three times a week, with occasional salt foot soaks as needed. After a few months, I stopped the salt foot baths, as they were no longer required.

I came to realise that there must be a reason for any setback, and I'd had a few. During the years of struggling alone, I had dismissed things causing me problems as not working, which wasn't the case. But I didn't know how to get them working for me. Now I learned to stop and examine things when setbacks occurred. Taking the time to see if I'd done anything differently helped to identify a reason. I could then address it and continue to move forward.

Books aided my understanding of the healing journey, and I tried to remember that self-encouragement was important. On days when my mood was low, Ian would sit with me and encourage me. He'd make lighthearted jokes about how glad we should be that this wasn't his journey, as he would have fallen at the first fence. And his shoulders were a huge cushion when tears overflowed.

A lifetime of demands on my time made it difficult to break the habit of pushing myself beyond my limits. Life also interrupts sometimes, and although I could deal with stress better overall, I could see that stress management needed more attention. I still felt something was holding me back physically.

It might be the last obstacle to overcome... if I could uncover what it was.

# Chapter 11

# Dietary Revelations

Since I got married, I always considered my diet to be healthy, but my journey back from cognitive issues taught me that my dietary choices didn't suit my body. A few months into wedded bliss, I presented with a condition thought to be rheumatoid arthritis (RA). Pain and stiffness in my upper limbs were so intense that Ian would put them through a range of movements before I could get going in the morning.

Holding a plate to serve the patients with meals at work was an effort, as any pressure on my joints was agony. Blood results, though, didn't support the diagnosis, but I knew from my nursing career that wasn't unusual. While blood tests such as erythrocyte sedimentation rate and c-reactive protein may indicate inflammation in the body, that's not always the case with around 40% of results being at normal levels.

There is no specific diagnostic test for RA, but the following tests may help reach a diagnosis. The rheumatic factor may show in 60-70% of cases and, if absent, a blood test for anti-citrullinated peptide (anti-ccp) may be helpful. Diagnosis is not by blood tests alone, but positive blood results are significant in the presence of other symptoms. Further investigations have to be conducted. Healthy individuals have shown these antibodies, while some people with autoimmune issues don't show the antibodies.

Some people can develop the antibodies later, but most do not. Other arthritic conditions have to be ruled out when there are no seropositive blood results. As my blood results were negative, treatment was ampoules of Calciferol, vitamin D2, rather than anti-rheumatic drugs. My brother Gerard had been allergy tested at the time and was allergic to many agents. As Calciferol didn't ease my pain, I treated it as a sensitivity to something and didn't return to the doctor.

I bought a book describing the issues from additives in the diet and set about removing them from mine. I changed to a high-fibre diet, and in around 18 months, I was pain-free. Over the years, the pain would recur, but blood results remained negative. This was my diet until the kids came along.

Another dietary change came with Dad's admission into long-term care because of Alzheimer's. Mad Cow Disease came to light in the UK in 1986, and variant Creutzfeldt-Jakob disease surfaced in the 1990s. My distress at his decline and his marked ataxic gait led my mind to make its own association. After blaming his illness on eating meat, I became a vegetarian.

My vegetarian diet was healthy, but that meant I ate a lot of grains and legumes. I remained vegetarian for ten years, only giving it up on feeling unwell for other reasons, but I carried a vegetarian mindset with me. There were plenty of vegetables on the dinner plate and a few plant-based meals a week.

I said I would share some of the private parts of my life, and in this instance, this relates to how our choices and environment affect us. Both dietary approaches are healthful. Yet another situation presented alongside rheumatoid arthritis for me, which I didn't consider could be linked at that time. It marked one of the darkest experiences of my life when, out of the blue, unannounced, and undoubtedly unwelcome, I displayed serious anger and rage issues.

## Warts and All

As painful as it is for me to revisit this time in my life, what I came to learn has helped me come to terms with it. I got married in 1982, and I can honestly say in the 24 years up till then, I'd never experienced rage before. And Ian and I had only ever had one disagreement in the years before we married.

But now, believe it or not, all 5ft of me couldn't get to my 6ft husband during these outbursts. He had the sense to get out of my way and stay barricaded behind a closed door to prevent the situation escalating beyond an argument.

I was distraught in the aftermath. But it felt like something was driving my behaviour, yet I couldn't put my finger on what. On searching for a reason, I eventually came up with one. I'd experienced a violent sexual assault in my teens, and although I'd had counselling, I had only scratched the surface. Perhaps the violence experienced was why I now acted like a madwoman, but I wasn't ready to deep dive into counselling again.

My diet moved away from a lot of wholegrain foods when the boys were young, due to their preferences, and I tried to stay calm. Things remained like this until I became a vegetarian, and the grain content of my diet rose again. The second time around, the rage was worse.

The rheumatoid arthritis presentation suggests I likely had a leaky gut back then. In my thirties, the ovarian cyst wreaked havoc in my tummy and might have contributed to more gut damage. Aggressive disorder can accompany leaky gut, but from all I discovered on this journey, my anger response seems to escalate to rage with a diet containing more grains.

Not knowing I was sensitive to gliadin, I did not know about its links to behavioural issues. And boy, did I love grains and bread. I learned this love is aided by a response that gluten causes, which keeps you going back for more. So it's no surprise that gluten intolerance might play a role in addiction to food and alcohol.

This replay of rage focused mainly on my son Adam, who I was trying to keep on the straight and narrow. He was lucky to have Ian and Simon to pull me off him – and that's not an exaggeration.

I've since read a lot about gliadin sensitivity and behavioural issues. But it would be good to have more public awareness of this, as I'd rather be gluten-free than a female version of the Incredible Hulk. I read of others who experienced emotional outbursts or rage episodes and regained their equilibrium on coming off gluten.

None of us want to hurt the people we love, and I wonder how many relationships have been ruined due to people being misunderstood. More so when dietary adjustments may help.

There would be more revelations to come as my education of a lifetime continued.

# Chapter 12

# More Changes Needed

As well as having to remove gluten from my diet, I discovered I may need to pay attention to the fats I consume due to the role of APoE4 in fat metabolism. The advised healthy fats don't always mix well with the APoE4 gene, so I was advised coconut oil has the potential to raise my cholesterol. I now cook with ghee or avocado oil and use olive oil for salad dressings and raw soups. I had to get over the fact that avocado oil is green in colour, but now there's always an extra bottle in my cupboard.

I won't bore you with the dental issues I've had, but they helped direct me to the work of Dr Weston Price. Dr Price studied the impact of diet on native communities and discovered that people eating the traditional way didn't succumb to what he called the "diseases of civilisation". But when they ate a Westernised diet of white flour and canned produce, they developed cavities and health issues.

The traditional diet consisted of high-fat meats, eggs, offal, whole grains, fruits, vegetables, and fermented foods. Correct food preparation was crucial, and made it more easily digestible. People also knew what foods aided fertility. Childbirth was more manageable, and those eating the traditional diet gave birth to healthier children.

The SNP on the MTHFR gene led me to look into diet again. While SNPs might have little effect and could even bring positive attributes by reducing my detox capacity, it was important to learn more.

On reading about suggested dietary support, I felt like running away. One of the best foods for a high folate intake is liver. I ate liver as a child, so it's not that I couldn't eat it. It was more that I didn't want to handle it.

Seafood was another recommendation. Ian had an incident with a fishbone in childhood, making him a very careful diner with fish. So I'd moved to frozen breaded fish now and then, reducing my intake. Thankfully, eggs are good. As I considered further dietary changes, "don't tell me" churned at the back of my head. I reread the information, hoping it was a joke. That "only kidding" would pop up somewhere, but no.

The Nutrigenetic Counsellor I saw through the clinic advised me that I would never get enough folate from vegetables – the first indication that my vegetarian days had not been one of my better decisions.

To support the SNP on the MTHFR gene, I should include wild fish, liver, and eggs, and on making such changes there were signs my ability to detox was improving. However, while things were progressing, at times I still felt myself going backwards physically. Omega-3 kept popping into my mind, but nothing stood out on doing internet searches.

My own previous research discovered several medical professionals who had come off a vegetarian diet because of ill health. I decided I had to find out why, and what they were suggesting. I still ate two vegetarian meals a week, sneaking a third if I felt I was eating enough fish and liver – often as pâté. But I could feel things weren't right. Perhaps continuing veggie meals was still not supporting my genetics enough for reasons I didn't yet know.

The writings of Dr Catherine Shanahan taught me that a genetic mutation doesn't mean the gene won't work. She also increased my understanding that I might be better on the traditional diet. During the years I struggled to stave off symptoms myself, I had joined a few health summits. That's where I'd first heard of Dr Terry Wahls.

Dr Wahls was in a wheelchair from secondary progressive Multiple Sclerosis, facing the reality that mainstream medicine couldn't help her. She took her health into her own hands and developed the Wahl's protocol! Within a year, she was walking with no walking aid, and the turnaround she achieved led me to read what she had to say. That's where I discovered what I needed to know about omega-3s.

Nutritionists advised me to eat organic to make my diet as clean as possible. I didn't know why grass-fed meat was preferable to grain-fed, but learned that meat from grain-fed animals has fewer omega-3s and more omega-6s. As the body can't make essential fatty acids, we need to supply them. People with autoimmune illnesses and brain conditions may have a greater fatty acid requirement, but a vegetarian diet lacks the omega-3 fatty acids we need for optimal function. It also leans more towards a higher level of omega-6, and higher consumption of omega-6 fatty acids can lead to inflammation in the body.

Meat also supplies all the amino acids we need, while a plant-based diet doesn't. Proteins from animal products are necessary for healing the gut if the digestive system is in a poor state. In contrast, a vegetarian diet may impede recovery and can reduce the amount of stomach acid we have. We need stomach acid for good digestion and what we absorb from food. I considered my diet might still not be optimal enough for my best chance of cellular healing.

## The MTHFR Gene

The MTHFR gene is involved with a process called methylation, which has a role in how healthy or ill we become, and it's involved with how genes express themselves. When this process isn't working well, there are genes you may prefer to be turned off that get turned on, and vice versa. In his book, Dirty Genes, Dr Ben Lynch describes this in detail.

The MTHFR may link to many health conditions, including Alzheimer's disease. A vegetarian diet doesn't supply all the essential nutrients for the MTHFR to work well, so it's advisable for vegans and vegetarians to supplement to ensure support of the methylation cycle. Omnivores who are not eating enough animal protein can also be deficient in B12, which will affect the MTHFR and the methylation cycle.

As mentioned, my cellular B12 levels were previously shown to be low, and although I was back to eating meat, it was only a small amount. But diet alone might not have been the only thing affecting methylation for me. A toxin build-up can also slow methylation down, and stress increases the demand for methylation. Both situations applied to me. For anyone needing to stay on a vegetarian diet, Dr Terry Wahls and Dr Catherine Shanahan give guidance through their books on doing that well to supply the body with what it needs.

As I read more about others who had regained health by including dietary measures, I learned that a high intake of vegetables and an intake of allowed fruits are also very important. I had to accept what diet was best for my genetic makeup and nutritional needs, but I had to get the balance right. My diet now contains a higher amount of fresh vegetable content than when I was a vegetarian, as grains are a thing of the past, and I've reduced legume intake. However, I can't afford to skimp on animal protein.

## Chapter 13

# Supported By Spirit

I llness interrupts the flow of our lives, making it difficult to attend to many things. Day-to-day necessities like making meals, household chores, and exercise can be too much, and may have a knock-on effect on our emotional wellbeing. As all our effort then goes into recovery, self-care, meditation, or spiritual practice (if participated in) may fall away. Exhaustion from trying to get well, and unknown physical issues taking shape in the background, meant keeping up a spiritual practice was too much for me at times. But I was supported as I worked at recovering my health, and I share this in gratitude.

I have always had my own beliefs because of things I've experienced. Such events are hard to deny when you're the one having them, but my parents were a little fearful of my experiences. Dad called me Gypsy Rosalee and convinced me no good would come of things I felt. So I developed nothing further.

Yet Spirit never leaves you; you only need to be present and open. Guidance, insights, and valuable premonitions have helped me through my darkest times. It was difficult getting time for myself when Mum was ill, but I found the Isis School of Holistic Health in Glasgow. I completed shamanic training, which nurtured my soul, and gave me a way where I feel comfortable with the spiritual helpers I've been aware of in my life.

The medium Angel Anne told me that the room I work from at home had an angelic presence, and I later received confirmation from Spirit in that very room. It was both loud and continuous until it got my attention and conveyed the most beautiful scent I have ever witnessed. And I wasn't alone. Ian also got to share in this beautiful experience.

It shouldn't have been a surprise then when I felt an angelic presence in my energy field. Yet, my Catholic upbringing at first convinced me it couldn't be so. The presence would give me numbers and told me to look them up as Angel Numbers. I did, and accepted the advice with gratitude. Such visits occurred in September 2018 when I realised I might have cognitive symptoms once more, and continued through to December 2020.

From the wealth of information the numbers gave, I took out what resonated with my situation. From the numbers 22 and 222, I felt I was to trust that the Angels and the Ascended Masters were guiding me. Have faith, remain positive, and things would work out in Divine timing. Number 43 reinforced this support. Later, when I was processing my mother wound, the number 11 brought advice to remove negativity and negative thoughts from my life, and to focus on the right things. Positive people and positive thoughts result in a positive impact. We might know that dredging up the past will gain nothing, but sometimes we just need reminding.

During this time, I received a reading from Debbie Clayton. I hadn't mentioned these angelic visits to anyone, but Debbie could tell me I was receiving them. She told me not to deny that I was getting information from Angels and, in my case, they would give me numbers. It was great to receive such confirmation. The last number from angelic presence was 7, received in December 2020. I felt the advice related to looking further into developing my spirituality.

Because of my health and the Covid restrictions on events, I joined an online course with the Isis School from October 2020, which let me take part at a level I could manage. The school later ran an ancestral healing course which coincided with my being restricted by physical problems. While I was finding it difficult to move forward, these community gatherings helped to carry me through and take part in spiritual practice when able.

## Nature Intelligence

Sometime previous to my second episode of cognitive issues, a wood nymph introduced herself to me during meditation. Nymphs are of the same proportion as humans. They are always female, and are considered divine spirits in partnership with nature. She informed me that her name was Aurelia, and I'm aware of her presence when she plays with my hair.

Before anyone thinks I'm away with the fairies, let me explain a little about nature intelligence. They are a significant part of the evolutionary path with the Deva Kingdom, comprising deva, nature spirits, elves, fairies, etc. Deva means "Being of Light" or "Shining One" in Sanskrit. Ancient races had reverence for this nature kingdom, seeing them as important as the human spirit. Theosophy corroborates that the Deva Kingdom exists.

The Deva Kingdom has a separate evolutionary path from us. However, their path runs alongside ours, with differences in how we develop. We grow through a route of Harmony Through

Conflict. It follows that our experiences may be painful, gaining wisdom through challenging life experiences. Deva grows through joy.

As part of the Divine plan, they are the intelligence behind nature but have many functions on planet earth, and the etheric world where they live permeates our world. Nature spirits may only be visible by those with an active third eye; however, people in touch with their sixth sense faculty may sense them. Civil engineer, author, clairvoyant, and artist, Eskild Tjalve explains that one of their roles is energy transmission during meditation and ceremonies, which may help you to understand my experience (noted in my journal below) as I tried to resume a meditation practice in 2018.

- - -

*In November 2018, as I prepared breakfast, an unseen force tousled my hair, so I allowed some time for meditation rather than postponing as I had planned. I sometimes journal during meditation time, but I put the pen down as my hair was being played with constantly. I asked Aurelia if she had something to tell me. As I experienced memory problems once more, my emotions were up and down.*

*The message was spirit was supporting me, and all was happening in its own time. Take one day at a time, and things would fall into place. She showed me a DNA strand and conveyed it was important for people to know individual biochemistry was important. She then communicated that we should recognise that individual detoxification pathways may be different, and genetics may play a role in that. So a pill won't fix everyone, and there's a need to take responsibility for our health. Then, she finished by relaying that I'm not the story. The route to recovery is.*

*As I entered meditation the next day, I recalled exposure to insecticide in the month before my mum's death. I then saw the inside of the shop in my mind's eye. It was an obvious message that something within the shop was contributing to my situation. Taking the blame for things comes easy to me, and my tendency to take the blame took over, recalling insecticide exposure before the shop opened.*

*It was my doing, and I didn't realise the dangers of toxin exposure. The level of heat affects some toxins in the atmosphere, and I kept the shop warm for remedial treatments. Could this have predisposed the very first neurological episode in 2011? Grateful there may be a reason for my experience, I left this meditation with a sense of peace.*

- - -

There is truly a feeling of this clairvoyant gift being a blessing when I look back at this. It was highlighting to me the shop rather than the insecticide, and this occurred a year before I had been forced to leave due to mould exposure. At the time, I had latched onto the insecticide perhaps being another reason for my symptoms; at that point, any reason gave me hope of being able to treat it.

Yet the message conveyed so much more that I had still to learn. This was several months before I found Dr Bredesen's book. I knew nothing of ReCODE and how individual biochemistry can play a role in symptoms. I knew nothing of detox pathways or that I had an SNP on the MTHFR gene that affected mine.

Any cause for my symptoms was welcome because their return frightened me, and a cause brought hope of treatment. However, Aurelia's message regarding biochemistry, detoxification, and genetics was far more significant than my knowledge at the time.

## Shamanic Helpers

I also received much support and guidance from the shamanic helping spirits, even if my health interrupted my connection. During a journey in April 2019, they advised I should look into the qualities of chillies and cayenne pepper as healers. I was also to support the pancreas, and I received healing at the solar plexus.

The pancreas support struck a chord because of the prediabetes, and I used essential oils for this. As for cayenne, according to clevelandclinic.org, chillies and cayenne can help a number of things, but the important one for me was improving digestion. I was by this point on the Gaps diet, as my digestion had been severely affected. I added cayenne, and later chillies, to bone broth and raw soups I made.

During an online course with the Isis School, I learned that you could ask the helping spirits for a healing dream. What a gift if I would only have used it in moderation! The first dream recommended tomatoes. I discovered that the tomato offers a few health benefits and is especially good for gut health. A prebiotic food, tomatoes help feed our gut bacteria and assist with how probiotics act in the intestine. This helps maintain a healthy balance in the microbiome, aiding it to work at its most optimal for us. This information moved me away from smoothies to making raw soups, both for the benefits and to reduce a tendency to prediabetes.

A second dream brought information on the herb basil. It's thought to benefit digestion and feed the healthy bacteria in our gut. Beneficial for tummy upsets, oils found across the various types of basil are anti-inflammatory. It also helps balance the pH level of the body. Other health benefits are thought to include management of diabetes and lowering cholesterol and triglyceride levels, and it may be helpful for depression. Its support of liver function and detoxification was a significant insight for me, as that was an area where I needed support. Basil leaves now go into many of the raw soups I make, and a basil and mint tea is among the range of herbal teas I'm able to drink.

I was on a roll. I asked for another healing dream and woke up to a voice telling me to look up mould implants. This led me to websites of ladies who had had breast implants which were affected by mould. I can only put what happened next down to my misplaced enthusiasm.

The website I read made it clear it was not a guide on how to recover. The author shared what had worked for her and stressed she didn't have SIBO or any gut issues. I believe the message I was supposed to get was that healing isn't linear, that I should relax, and let things unfold (and stop bothering the helping spirits for a healing dream for a while).

But I didn't get that. Enthusiasm is a substantial driving force, and I latched onto something that wasn't a good idea for me. It's almost embarrassing to admit, but the website author had found a garlic oil that had helped her dog's ear infections. So I thought I would try it for mine. In fairness, I'd tried to treat my ears for seven years by this point.

I took the garlic drops orally. By good fortune, my clinic appointment was soon after. It turned out that garlic oil could be bad for my gut condition. I'd only been taking it for about one week and felt no obvious gut issues, but I had experienced some brain fog and slight problems with recall. Knowledge of the gut-brain axis helped me to realise that I was probably responsible for causing these symptoms. So, the garlic oil stopped there and then. I became very upset with myself, but it was also a valuable turning point.

Some months previously, the setback from walking had led me to make a shamanic journey for guidance. My helping spirits showed me I was taking myself around in circles. I was always pushing myself, and it was time to stop and support the gene that was brought to my attention. I also did a shamanic exercise to communicate with my body, and my journal entry read:

> *My body showed me I am forever focused on healing it, trying whatever way is needed to heal it. This was too much, in as much as my focus was too intent on this area. My body needs me to realise that while such healing is important, it wants me to rest more. Adequate sleep, rest throughout the day, and a reduction from stress.*

I'd already been informed of this, yet I was still focusing on healing, exhausting myself, and creating further setbacks. Tears flowed as I considered my actions with the garlic oil foolish, and questioned why I'd been so stupid. As I cried, I realised it wasn't impatience that kept me pushing myself on my quest for a return to health. It was fear. The years I'd battled against cognitive symptoms and lost had left me fearful that perhaps there was no solution.

But I now knew differently, emerging from a cognitive cloud having found ReCODE. It was time to relax and enjoy recovery happening in the here and now. I could go with the flow and work with my body. There was no longer any need to worry. I had still to uncover what was holding me back physically, but pushing myself had taken my attention away from that.

After this, things flowed more easily, and I felt guidance kept coming, steering me in the right direction. On another shamanic journey in June 2021, the helping spirits gave me the number 2 and told me to look it up as an angel number. The message was that I was to have courage, faith, and trust in the Angels and Universal energies. The answers to prayers were manifesting, although it might not be obvious just then.

Things did start to manifest the following month, but I didn't handle it right. It was the start of the ultimate obstacle I had to overcome.

## A Final Hurdle

Things unfolded in July 2021, which I didn't handle correctly for a few reasons. Perhaps the main one relates to the original misdiagnosed ovarian cyst, which was a long, drawn-out catastrophe that took years to resolve. It caused me to feel that I need to be certain if something needs medical attention, rather than risk a doctor making a mistake. While I don't aim to neglect myself, my need for certainty could have inadvertently meant I have.

We were also emerging from the restrictions of the second Covid lockdown, and there was continued advice not to overwhelm the NHS. I woke in the night with what felt like colic and went back to sleep, only to awaken later feeling as if spasms accompanied the colic. I got up to assess my situation and consider if it was something I should act upon, and decided against doing so. Initially, I didn't think anything major was wrong.

I don't have irritable bowel, but the fact that I was repeatedly given that diagnosis when an ovarian cyst was wreaking havoc in my gut, didn't help my decision. My mind made its own connections. Colic plus spasms equals a possible diagnosis of irritable bowel, so I decided to see if I could get it to settle down myself. It settled over the following two days, but my decision was still a mistake.

Symptoms arose over the following weeks, and I finally sought a doctor's advice (I know, after the horse had bolted). I was advised it might have been a leak of some sort, but by then there were no symptoms of concern. I felt angry at myself that I hadn't acted at the time, but on chatting to my son Simon, he agreed that I could hardly be blamed, based on my previous experience.

So after telling myself off, I tried to learn from this, and it alerted me to the importance of another pain which built up in February 2022. The impact of Covid-19 meant only telephone consultations were available with the doctor, so I phoned, recounting the previous incident and my genuine concern that another "leak" was going to happen. I also tried to convey that I might have an infection in my gut (due to mould) – to no avail. As for a diagnosis, let's just say irritable bowel was mentioned and prescribed for, with the addition of an anti-fungal because I mentioned infection. And it was downhill from there.

There was no acute pain, just a slow build-up. Doctors assisted me over further phone consultations, but unfortunately in the wrong direction. Four weeks later, the area of concern did give way to something, and it left me in chronic pain. Various referrals followed, and Covid's impact on hospital appointments complicated matters further.

I eventually found myself help, and surgery took place in November, but the damage was widespread. There was no doubt something had happened, but as it was now eight months down the line from the incident, I'll never know what that was. As mentioned, mycotoxins can colonise in the gut, leading to infection. Their immunosuppressant effects can also lead to dormant infections coming to the surface. I'll never know if either explanation was at the root of this, but it is a possibility.

## Chapter 14

# Insight Gained

While I gave my all to recovery, I couldn't truly move on until what was going on in my abdomen was attended. It was a physical stress on my body and standing in my way of further healing.

I'd done my best to stay on the supplements I could tolerate while awaiting medical attention, but nausea interfered as did a poor appetite. Pain interrupted my sleep and decreased my ability to exercise and so sticking to the protocol I'd been following was affected. Analgesia I was taking would be worsening leaky gut, and I did what I could to lessen the damage. As things worsened, I felt inflammation was occurring in my abdomen, and I knew all of the above could affect my cognitive health.

Familiar symptoms reappeared by the time I got doctors who would help me. Dizziness returned with mild headaches and pain in the area where something had whipped across the left side of my brain. I was acutely aware that cognitive health would be affected further if this went on much longer. My initial reluctance for surgery had faded because of this, and I was grateful to have arrived at the point where a diagnostic laparoscopy would be done.

Post-op recovery wasn't easy, as mobility was difficult and I couldn't lie flat at first, so sleep continued to be interrupted. I felt slower cognitively, which I regarded as linked to what had been going on in my gut and initially didn't consider that I'd also been unable to follow some of the protocol recommended for me. Symptoms I felt were related to mycotoxins had returned during this and I wondered if they may be involved somehow.

On trying to return to exercise and dietary measures to help further, things weren't going to plan. Each time I tried to push ahead, my gut spasmed and not only left me immobile but also unable to eat, so I was sabotaging my progress. Patience was necessary, and I began looking to see what I could do to help rather than hinder myself.

Attention to healing the gut continued. I took a short membership of the Wellness Plus website to learn if there was anything else I could do to help, and began doing a castor oil rub the evenings before the days I did a sauna. The oil was to be kept on overnight and was useful for anyone prone to adhesions. It also supports the liver in detoxing, and I could tell something was moving, leading to restarting Epsom salt foot baths occasionally and increasing saunas to three times a week.

There is a support group for APoE4 carriers and carers which I'd felt too unwell to join before, and on joining, a Support Team Intern welcomed me. I noticed her qualifications included ReCODE 2.0 Trained Health Coach – a term I'd never heard of – reminding me that research would have continued.

This led to my reading Dr Bredesens' book, The End of Alzheimer's PROGRAMME, where I learned of the additional subtypes discovered. I did feel a bit overwhelmed as I read the book, but reminded myself that as individuals we don't have all the predisposing factors. So, all of the content would not necessarily apply to me.

The book brought reassurance I wasn't imagining the cognitive slowness. It advised people who had gained improvement on the protocol may experience a setback because of infection. In addition, anaesthetics can be involved in cognitive decline for several reasons. And if antibiotics are given in the post-operative phase, they affect the gut flora as well. I could only wonder if these factors were also contributing to the cognitive slowness I felt.

While I could see it was clearing, I'd learned by now those senior moments we dismiss may be red flags. On returning from the hospital, I'd open a kitchen cupboard to put the milk away instead of the fridge. On entering a room, I'd sometimes need to stop and think about why I was in there. I would also sometimes need to take a moment to connect to my train of thought. These episodes passed in minutes, and I knew the milk didn't go into the cupboard, but I knew better than to ignore them.

## Baby Steps

As I love yoga, I planned to incorporate this into my self-care. But gut spasms halted my attempts, so this had to be shelved meantime as I respected my limits.

A hidden gem surfaced when restricted by ill health. The ability to distract myself by flinging myself into work projects or exercise wasn't possible, and at a deeper level, this experience of illness had changed me. Being housebound, the reality of my previous coping strategies was obvious. They had an important role, as they had helped get me through life. But they weren't always healthy. My mindset had changed. I no longer wanted to push myself beyond what I can do comfortably.

In the past, meditation was an essential part of my being and its missed effect always palpable, but this regular practice was long gone. Whether the effect from previous years of stress, or the effect of mycotoxins, or both, I'd been functioning on high alert for some time. I didn't know where to start in terms of stress management.

I introduced essential oils into my day to help balance my hormones. Oils were rubbed into the soles of my feet, which have many reflex points, attempting to reduce cortisol. I placed wooden diffusers in the bathroom with balancing oils. My workspace also had a wooden diffuser, and I used any additional oils I felt may be helpful, dependent on my mood. I also put a diffuser in my car to benefit from the oils when driving.

This illness interrupted my first attempt at reading Coming Home by Fi Sutherland, one of the teachers at the Isis School of Holistic Health. On returning to it, it was a valuable guide to learning to sit with myself. I had to become the observer of my world as, without realisation, there could be no change. I created a small notebook containing the advice from the book that was helpful to me. As things arose, I could refer to it and follow Fi's suggestions. I added a mindfulness app to my phone and acquainted myself with mindfulness practices. And my "go to" helper, the Bach remedies, were reintroduced.

A further measure of self-forgiveness came from reading The End of Alzheimer's PROGRAMME. Dr Bredesen writes how relationships may be affected long before cognitive symptoms present. It's known the progression of dementia starts years before, and he'd considered arguments in the home and elsewhere, and problems with mood, may be the initial signs of neurodegenerative illness long before diagnosis can be established.

I'd wondered about that, mainly when considering the aggression experienced which mystified me. But emotions ran in the background of my life outwith the aggression. I've spent much of this lifetime trying to overcome this with counselling for trauma experienced, to exhaustive examination of my relationship with my mum through various healing therapies.

While I surmised I've had leaky gut since way back in my early twenties, my inability to cope less well presented about five years after the problems with the ovarian cyst. I can only wonder if further damage to my gut increased my anxiety and reduced my ability to cope with stress.

With the exception of stressors outwith my control, one benefit this journey has brought me is I have never felt as calm in a long time. I've also recognised this person who's returned, and I haven't had the pleasure of her presence since my mid-teens.

## Time to Move on

I had read recommendations in The End of Alzheimer's PROGRAMME and considered what to do next. Mycotoxin levels needed to be reassessed, as did my gut issues and blood results for cholesterol, blood glucose and cortisol levels. While cognition was improving, I wanted advice. The book also touched upon self-help as well as finding help, and I checked the Apollo Health website.

On considering the best way forward, I learned of ReCODE 2.0 Certified Health Coaches, who helped support UK clients. The Apollo Health website explained the training of ReCODE 2.0 Health Coaches increased the help that could be offered to clients. I reached out to a Health Coach for help with the rest of this journey. Telemedicine means distance is not a problem, and it was time to get back in the saddle and continue to move forward.

I received a clarity call to discuss my concerns and we were good to go. The health coach liaised with a practitioner on my behalf, that led to my being helped to transition onto the ketoFLEX 12/3 way of eating recommended on the protocol. My food choices were pretty similar from all I'd learned, and the health coach thought it may not take too many tweaks to get me into ketosis.

Not only do ketones benefit the brain, but when all the advice is used together, metabolism and insulin sensitivity improves, inflammation may reduce, and autophagy can help remove beta-amyloid. It can also encourage detoxing, so for me, this contains many of the factors I need to restore my health. Again, everyone is different, so the ketoFLEX 12/3 will be individually tailored and can be vegetarian or include animal protein.

As the coach also worked alongside other practitioners, she was able to refer me to a practitioner for any necessary tests and protocol advice. At this point I made another discovery. The genetic information I had from the SelfDecode DNA Wellness report was for my information and clearly stated it did not include all the SNPs available. The Health Coach advised that there was more to it than the APoE4 and MTHFR that I knew about and I should again access my genetic raw data and apply for an Imputed Complete Gene Mutation Report. This was more useful to her, and the practitioner would go through the report with me.

My protocol was added to with a few additional supplements. The imputed gene report highlighted of fourteen genes involved with detoxification, five of mine had SNPs on both allele. The practitioner said this would be regarded as critical. Further testing would help throw light on whether more advice was needed in this area.

On receiving those results methylation was reported to be fine. There had been some areas of improvement with homocysteine levels reducing from 8.4 to 5.6. While 8.4 may not be regarded as too high, high homocysteine levels increase the risk for some diseases including dementia. Detoxification would need some support. Mycotoxin results showed the Mycophenolic Acid toxin had cleared and Ochratoxin A had reduced further. However, two other problems appeared. Enniatin B, a fungus mainly caused by water damaged buildings although it has been found in grains, and Gliotoxin. Gliotoxin is released by Aspergillus mould to hinder the immune system.

I felt I had to consider where to go from here. Working with the health coach was a good idea. While I was still in need of medical attention from mainstream medicine, the medical help received and the support of the health coach helped me to continue to move forward. I was managing the ketoFLEX diet, exercising daily, decluttering my personal space of items that had accumulated during the experience of cognitive decline. I had returned to personal shamanic practice, occasional meditation and replaced essential oils with somatic exercises which I found relaxed the nervous system.

Many functional practitioners talk about finding the root cause behind a person's ill health and I wondered if my healing efforts should look into further management of the mycotoxins. I knew of Dr Shoemaker's protocol for treating mould illness and visited the website survivingmold.com to see if any practitioner worked internationally with patients. To my surprise there was a practitioner in the UK who, having also trained with Dr Bredesen, would be able to advise me on ReCODE if needed.

# Chapter 15

# A New Way of Being

Mycotoxins were the main contributor to cognitive decline this time for me, and some may feel exposure to mould is rare and so less of a concern. However, there are many toxins that stockpile in our body that we may not be getting rid of.

Having succumbed to a toxic illness, I had to make many changes. Safe cleansing agents around the home were a must. Besides inhaling the chemicals in cleansing products, anti-bacterial cleaners also harm our microbiome. Dr Ben Lynch lists sprays and cleaners as some products that help make our genes dirty. Evidence also suggests that as well as the damage antibacterial and antimicrobial cleansers may lead to, warm water and soap or detergents do the job just as well.

Soda crystals, liquid soda crystals, bicarbonate of soda, citric acid, liquid soap, vinegar, and hydrogen peroxide have replaced the chemical cleaners I used before. I use Faith Canter's bleach recipe, and when recovering from surgery I learned of Nancy Birtwhistle's books, which gave me some more handy tips.

I have successfully used soap nuts and eco egg for laundry, but currently use Dri-Pak Liquid soap or Ecover laundry liquid. I was putting Epsom salts in as fabric conditioner for everything except towels, and using Ecover fabric conditioner for them. However, vinegar is a water softener on its own and I've found it works well with towels when added to the washing machine drum and fabric dispenser. Vinegar can be used as a stain remover for clothes, and the Friendly Soap brand of kitchen soap can be used for laundry stains.

For the dishwasher, it's Ecover dishwasher tabs. I refill hand soap containers with Dri-Pak liquid soap or use Method hand soap. And I now use an E-cloth deep clean mop for floors. You only need water when using E-cloths, so it means no harsh chemicals.

## Personal Care

I also had to change the personal care products and makeup I use. Some companies are doing their best to sell safe items, but they can include some less desirable ingredients, so it's necessary to read the labels. A link between titanium oxide in cosmetics and lung cancer has been suggested. This applies more to the powdered products, as it's inhaled.

I have used safe shower gels, but moved on to Friendly Soap, and I use their shea butter soap for my face. I do find the winter weather can dry out my skin since returning to soap, so I now include facial oils at times as well as creams, and the oils help with that. Dri-Pak liquid soap is approved for personal care use, and it can be used as a shower gel and shampoo.

Friendly Soap also do shampoo soaps and conditioner. I've had a continual amount of slight hair shedding throughout this journey, so my hair is much finer than before. I wondered if it was hormonal when it started, but later learned hair loss can be associated with leaky gut, and mould itself can cause hair loss if affected. For that reason, my hair gets more expensive products, and I use Champo products at present and Lanza Silver Brightening Shampoo.

I order make-up from MG Naturals, which are titanium oxide-free. Aluminium-free deodorants I mainly buy for Ian, and I may use them on an odd occasion.

To avoid overuse of over-the-counter or prescription medication, I use homoeopathy at home, Schuessler tissue salts, and essential oils for minor ailments. Guidance is needed with homoeopathy, but courses are available advising on how to do this. Essential oils need to be used with caution, so again advice for safe use is necessary.

## Cooking and Food Storage

I initially purchased Vision glass pots, however, I have read they can explode. I haven't experienced this, but two did get chipped, and I couldn't get the same size. I have an Xtrema casserole and a pot. This cookware retains the heat, and you can reduce the temperature once cooking is underway. I also have a small and a large slow cooker, and use glass or enamel dishes in the oven.

A carbon steel frying pan replaced a nonstick frying pan for me at first and I took care of the seasoning, cleaning, and reseasoning of it. I did eventually buy a green frying pan for Ian. This is ceramic nonstick, and the aluminium core is between stainless-steel, so theoretically it's safe for me to use as long as the ceramic coating doesn't get chipped. However, the health coach introduced me to Tefal Ingenio pots and pans which are stainless steel only and their frying pans are titanium nonstick, which helped make life easier.

I store some food in glass dishes. Stasher bags are used at times, mainly if I have some raw vegetable that I've cut and only used half, as I find it keeps well in a stasher bag. Russbe reusable freezer bags and Lakeland BPA-free freezer bags, are what I've used for freezing items, and I'm considering stojo freezer safe storage to save costs in the long term. Baking paper replaces aluminium foil, and I use silicone or wooden cooking utensils for the cookware, but have a few stainless-steel utensils.

## Lowering Costs

Major changes can be expensive and, as I'd been trying to fend off symptoms for so long, I initially jumped in feet first once I knew what was going on. That meant I spent more than I needed to, and in hindsight it would be fine to have gone at a slower pace.

I get meat delivered from organic farms that do a rewards scheme and, dependent on spend, free delivery. I also buy organic meat and other produce from Sainsburys and Waitrose, nitrate-free bacon, and organic vegetables where possible. Sainsbury's and Waitrose have a good organic range across their store, Asda has a fair selection of organic vegetables, and Marks and Spencer also offer some organic vegetables and meat. Lidl has organic vegetables and eggs, and I regularly buy their organic produce; they also have grass-fed beef. I use the reward schemes these stores offer.

As the health coach assisted transitioning onto the ketogenic diet a wider range of vegetables had to be included. It became clear buying organic had also constricted my diet as there were only certain organic vegetables available. So I had to let go of an organic only mindset and moved to organic where possible, and revisited farm shops in our area. There is also a list called the dirty dozen, which is available from the Pesticide Action Network UK and the Environmental Working Group US. This is a list of the vegetables and fruits which you can avoid, and choose varieties that are not on the list if organic vegetables aren't possible.

While I have made fermented foods, I allow myself the luxury of buying a good brand. They're a fair part of my diet, so I feel I'm worth the treat. Again, I use a company that offers rewards and free delivery, dependent on spend and stock up.

On introducing fish again, I initially got a fresh fish delivery. However, Ian isn't a great lover of fish, although he'll enjoy a small amount. To accommodate this, and the fact that in Scotland fresh salmon is farmed rather than wild caught, I now buy packs of frozen wild caught fish. This proves good value for money for me, and the portions are a good size for Ian.

While he eats what I cook, he doesn't give up the snacks and foods that he likes, so we buy him some organic ready meals to ensure he doesn't feel he's missing out. I try to do meal planning, because if I'm organised with meals there's less waste, and leftovers are useful for lunches. Pinterest is handy for pinning recipes I want to try on boards, and I tidy them up now and then. I also shop more as I need things, again to reduce waste.

As mentioned, personal care includes Friendly Soap, which I find very economical. At present, I find Dri-Pak products value for money, and Wilko also sell their brand of some of the products. I've started to get vinegar in bulk from Amazon and I shop around, which means visiting a few supermarkets. But if I plan, it's doable.

## My Keystone Moments

This has not been an easy road. Mould exposure can be devastating on the body, and my recovery from that continues, but I no longer have balance issues and, with the exception that recent illness slowed me down cognitively, I don't have the cognitive symptoms I had at the start.

There was a lot to change, and it wasn't easy initially, having a sense of panic due to attempting to ward off cognitive symptoms for so long. There were tears at times when I felt overwhelmed, or from the crazy thoughts due to mycotoxins. But there were some lighthearted moments along the way. The situations that brought them about were not ones I thought would ever raise a smile.

I did the Hulda Clark parasite cleanse because I tested positive for a parasite with the Field Control Therapy. While I couldn't stretch to reading books about parasites in food, for fear I'd never eat again, I did try some suggested practices I came across. One involved using public toilets, so one day while out shopping on my own, when the need arose I decided to perch above the toilet seat in a public convenience. The damp rim around both hems of my trousers ensured I would never do that again.

While I was a reluctant enema user, they were needed. I organised the enema bag on a coat hanger, and used a clothes airer to place the hanger on. One day, as I lay on the floor beside a bed in our spare room, ready for action, the clothes airer started to topple. I just managed to stop the contents from going all over me, and my expletives had Ian running to my assistance. I screamed in my frustration, warning him to enter the room in fear of his life. As he checked I was okay from the other side of the door, little did I know I might come to regret not letting him in.

That came when I tried my hand at contrast showers. People who know me well will find it laughable that I've ever stood under a cold shower, as I'm famously known as being "cauld riffed". And my first attempt was unsuccessful. As I jumped from hot to cold, front of body to back of body, the shower mat creased up and I took a header towards the shower screen, knocking it off the wall.

I did of course scream as I hurled towards the screen, and as I lay, with my arm jammed between the bath and the bottom of the screen, I wondered why Ian hadn't come to my aid. Emerging wounded – more emotionally than physically – I went downstairs to ask if he had actually heard me scream. He had, but apparently he'd thought I was just screaming because the water was cold.

Last but not least, it goes without saying that my periods of rage caused me distress, both at the time and in recalling them later. I felt shame and guilt about these episodes, as my sons suffered in this madness. So, finding out there was a cause doesn't allow me to condone them. However, on discovering there was a reason driving such behaviour as I initially thought, I will leave this world at peace.

I've cried over this many times, and once I'd discovered what had gone on, I got it all off my chest during a chat with Ian one day. Tears flowed but broke into a smile as Ian, ever my rock, told me, "I knew there was something really wrong with you, love, I truly did. I knew someone who could be so loving would not naturally act like that, and I thought it must be the menopause." What can I say? Western society certainly gives the menopause a bad press.

Part Three

## I Have Learned

# Chapter 16

# Dietary Confusion

I t's no wonder we're confused, with all the conflicting advice surrounding diet. Don't have salt. Reduce egg consumption. Fats are bad, etc. Various dietary advice has left us not knowing what is best for our health. But in having to address my diet, I've learned that some of this is misinformation and can be detrimental to health.

The promotion of a low-fat diet has raised questions, because not everyone agrees the diet is beneficial. Senator George McGovern supported its introduction and gave no attention to the concerns of scientists who opposed it. No proof supported the ideas behind it to be valid, and the arguments over its benefits have continued to this day. Despite its promotion, ill health continues to increase.

We should have salt in our diet, although it should be sea salt. Dr Catherine Shanahan writes that salt improves digestion, energy levels, learning and concentration, and bone health. It improves the taste of food, reduces hunger, and can help in reversing insulin resistance and diabetes.

Without a doubt, the outcome of consuming an inadequate diet can be damaging to us. Consider putting petrol into a diesel car, or vice versa; the vehicle no longer performs at its best and can totally break down. I had to accept that the food I chose as fuel for my body had to change a little once more. Gluten had gone. For me the MTHFR gene needs what animal protein brings to my body, and the APoE4's role in fat metabolism and transport means I need to be using the right type of fats. Dr Terry Wahls explains that food is not a cure-all, but diet can bring improvement. The important insight I've gained is that dietary choices should be tailored to our individual needs. Bioindividual nutrition is thought to have a role in healthcare in the future in functional medicine.

The major culprit is the processed diet. Our fast-paced lives have led us to favour convenience foods and removed us from the fact that, at a basic level, we are still a species. A species that performs at its optimal level when it's getting everything it needs, and that includes what we eat. If we keep taking in bad fuel, the resultant reduction in performance or eventual breakdown our body gets from it may manifest as illness.

As well as giving food a longer shelf-life, processing is aimed at making the consumer want more. I'm thinking of my bread binges again as I write this. We fill our supermarket trolley, but it's not at the forefront of our mind that we're also buying the chemical additives the food contains. It follows that our bodies have to get rid of such chemicals.

The processed diet can also encourage inflammation. Low-level inflammation is related to being overweight, and chronic inflammation can be the impetus behind many diseases. To quote Dr Dale Bredesen: "If you want to give yourself Alzheimer's? Stick to the processed diet."

## Epigenetics

It's been thought that the diseases we can develop were down to variants in the DNA, but epigenetics changes that.

Epigenetics is the study of how our genes express themselves as a result of our behaviours and environmental factors, and as external contributors play a role, we can turn gene expression around. One of the main contributors influencing epigenetics is the diet we eat.

While gene expression is not down to diet alone, it has a significant role. How much exercise we get, toxin exposure, and stress are other factors affecting gene expression. If established, such changes in gene expression pass on to our children and, research has shown, even to grandchildren.

The study of epigenetics shifts the focus to understanding that some of the diseases we develop are related to our behaviours and environmental circumstances, giving us some choice in how our genes behave.

# Chapter 17

# We Live in a Toxic World

Modern society has exposed us to many environmental toxins which are difficult to avoid, harming us silently as we remain unaware. They flood our system through the air we breathe, absorption through the layers of our skin and what we ingest, building up in the body, creating a foundation for disease. Many toxins are carcinogenic, and our bodies can't process and remove such a toxic burden.

## The War on Plastic

The impact of plastic on the environment is a concern, and it's a concern for our well-being, too. Canned food is lined with plasticisers, and food and drink containers made from plastic omit phthalates into the products they contain. This includes baby formula bottles, if made of plastic. Personal care items in plastic containers, and detergents for home use, carry the same risk. So avoidance can be very difficult.

They are endocrine disruptors affecting our hormonal system and the brain, and a buildup in the cells can lead to triggers for cancer. Guidance may state small amounts are harmless, for example, in a small bottle of water. However, accumulated load may be tremendous depending on how much water we consume, or from eating food purchased in plastic packaging, and from other sources.

It's known that oestrogen can cause breast cancer cells to proliferate. When scientists witnessed breast cancer cells in test tubes increase, they discovered it was due to the phthalates from the test tubes that contained them. The plasticiser's effect on breast tissue was similar to oestrogen. Phthalates stockpiling in the body may contribute to hormone-affected tumours.

## A Breath of Fresh Air

Smoke flowing from industrial chimneys carries dioxins and other poisons into the atmosphere. They descend on our waterways and soil, and we absorb them through the skin and by inhalation. There is pollution from automobile exhausts, and we might inhale fumes from petrol or diesel as we refill the tank of a car.

Fumes from furnishings, carpets, and fire-retardant applications on furnishings accumulate in our homes. Paints, turpentine, wallpaper pastes, or glues from wallboard all emit fumes. Bleach, laundry detergents, and anti-bacterial sprays are all chemicals and detrimental to us when stockpiled in our bodies.

Scented candles are another source of toxins. They emit limonene, formaldehyde, petroleum distillates, esters, and alcohol. Once the paraffin wax burns, it gives off benzene, toluene, and acetone. These chemicals are carcinogenic and cause allergies and skin issues. They can also precipitate asthma attacks.

Soot from the burning candle affects the air quality, reaching the bloodstream after being inhaled through the lungs. This can contribute to respiratory disease, strokes, and heart attacks. Fragrance may also pose a problem as synthetically produced fragrance gives off volatile chemicals that can be detrimental to health.

Safe alternatives are soy candles or beeswax candles. Beeswax candles can help clean the indoor air quality as they release negative ions.

## Water, Water Everywhere

But is it safe to drink? Do you consider how contaminated your tap water is at home? How many chemicals are going into your cup of tea? While it's necessary to remove microorganisms from the water supply, studies have linked chlorine to tumour formation and arteriosclerosis. Contaminants can gather from pipes as water travels from treatment plants to your home. Herbicides and pesticides get into the water supply, and chemical treatments may not remove them all. Accidental spillage and seepage of pesticides through the soil can occur, which can affect the endocrine system. Potential outcomes are alterations in puberty onset in children, infertility issues, and breast and prostate cancer.

Drugs get into the water from urine, giving a continual supply of substances we don't need through drinking water. Even well-diluted drug residues can affect human cell function. Oestradiol is oestrogen from the contraceptive pill, found in 80% of water sites tested, and this may interfere with the balance of sex hormones in developing children. In addition, more males may develop gynecomastia, and it may affect the prostate gland and human fertility.

There's a suggested association between aluminium and fluorine in drinking water and dementia, because fluorine can raise the amount of aluminium absorbed. A study carried out by researchers from the University of Edinburgh and Stirling University in Scotland showed dementia risk rose where water contained natural levels of fluoride and higher aluminium levels. At the time of writing, there is no added fluoride in Scotland's water. The study stated:

"Higher levels of aluminium and fluoride were related to dementia risk in a population of men and women who consumed relatively low drinking water levels of both."

Similar studies supported this link, while others did not. The larger the study, the more prone results were to show a link between aluminium levels and dementia risk. In the words of the researchers involved in the study in Scotland, "This suggests that there may be no safe levels of these substances when it comes to dementia risk."

## Mirror, Mirror on the Wall

What goes on the skin can go through the skin, making some shampoos, skin care products, and cosmetics a hazard we should avoid. We also inhale fumes from cologne, deodorants, nail varnish, and nail varnish remover. Some children's products contain formaldehyde and dioxane – a known carcinogen. Mineral oil, derived from petroleum, is in some baby products. In Europe, mineral oil use depends on its passing purity regulations to meet adequate safety levels, which may not be so elsewhere. Exposure to such toxins from birth has the potential to affect a child's development.

Aluminium in antiperspirants reaches the sweat glands and stops perspiration. It has been found in breast cancer tissue, highlighting that the body isn't getting rid of it all. Dr Clair Bailey wrote an article in the Mail on Sunday's 'You' magazine in which she explained that a study looking at the concentration of aluminium in breast tissue suggested the metal can accumulate when there is frequent use of deodorants with aluminium. The study suggested a frequency of use, plus the younger the age when use starts, may make a person more liable to develop breast cancer. Antiperspirants are the most common route of aluminium exposure.

I discovered late in my recovery that a mascara I was buying from a cosmetic company marketing their products as safe, actually contained aluminium. And a well-known brand of Epsom salts I purchased contained EDTA; it defeats the purpose of detoxing if I'm soaking in a bath with EDTA added.

While EDTA itself doesn't absorb through the skin, it's a known penetration enhancer, yet it is reported as safe by the Cosmetic Review Panel. It affects the skin surface in a way that allows other chemicals and ingredients through. Added to a bath, EDTA helps other ingredients in the bath salts, plus any metals from the tap water, to get into the system. I now always check the labels.

Biopsies have shown toxins accumulate in fat cells in our body and don't just stay there. They seep out, damaging our health and speeding up ageing.

## On Today's Menu

Plastic is polluting oceans, affecting sea life and plants. Industrialisation emissions descend on our waterways and soil, leading to heavy metals getting into the food chain. Systemic pesticides may affect crops, as they can be fully absorbed by the plant rather than just affect the surface of the produce alone. Unfortunately, food washing or peeling is often not enough to prevent exposure.

And let's not forget the additives, colourings, and preservatives present in the processed diet. Polystyrene containers for takeaway food and drinks allow exposure to styrene, which is a known carcinogen. Each sip of coffee or tea through a takeaway cup may be introducing microplastics into your system.

## Aluminium

The debate surrounding aluminium and health continues and so it's worth mentioning on its own. Studies show that small amounts of repeated exposure may be toxic to us, especially for children and the developing embryo. The number of avenues for exposure is vast, from aluminium food containers and foil, cooking utensils, pots, makeup, and personal care products. It's also more likely to contaminate acidic food and drinks in canned produce and canned drinks.

Antacids and other medications can contain aluminium. The Spinal Centre of Australia's website describes aluminium as a neurodegenerative poison, and advises:

"No living systems use aluminium as part of a biochemical process. Without stating the obvious, it is not part of the food chain. So to be blunt, stop eating, drinking, bathing, spraying, and cooking in aluminium. Be careful."

A known neurotoxin, researchers suspect it has a role in ALS, Parkinsonism, and Alzheimer's disease, although you may find information to the contrary on some Alzheimer's websites.

It can cross the blood-brain barrier in some people. However, factors related to aluminium make examination of its toxicity problematic, so confirming a definite connection is difficult.

I later showed aluminium in my blood and had to take steps to remove it. This was a surprise, as I'd never used antiperspirants containing aluminium since my late twenties. Aluminium cooking pots, utensils, and baking foils were no longer used, and I thought I'd removed other sources from 2013, having experienced cognitive decline. Some aluminium that showed up might have already been in my cells and mobilised with the detoxing methods used for the mycotoxins.

But, without thinking, I was exposing myself to aluminium through the occasional takeaway delivered in a foil container. I drank draught lager before coming off gluten, then draught cider, and didn't know draught beers were stored in aluminium barrels.

The debate on whether aluminium has a role in Alzheimer's disease remains ongoing. Previous arguments against its involvement were back in the 1990s. However, as studies show more about the neurotoxicity of aluminium, it warrants being considered for further research.

# Chapter 18

# The Changing Face of Medicine

I t's impossible to know how our forebears understood health and disease. One assumption is that they learned the value of various plants by trial and error. However, superstition accompanied serious illness and death, and treatments aimed to undo the supernatural forces at work. Progression from a superstition to a scientific standpoint in medicine took a while, and Hippocrates helped move illness out of the supernatural realm.

He supported natural cure and the lesser use of drugs, viewing the patient holistically within his environment. His belief was that the body could heal and restore itself. His approach was both clinical and natural, seeing lifestyle, diet, environmental factors, and inherited factors as contributors to disease. Humorist theory may have begun in Ancient Egyptian medicine, but Greek scholars and doctors arranged it into an organised system. It's believed Hippocrates developed the theory of the humors further, and it influenced medicine for two thousand years.

It was also a move away from superstition. Physicians could differentiate between illnesses, and note-taking assisted clinical observation. A view of illness developed, combining environmental factors and the body's internal terrain.

The Black Death in the fourteenth century brought destruction and no guidelines for addressing it. The death toll was immense, and the medical view, with emphasis on cause and prevention and minimal drug use, came to be seen as a handicap. Criticism of the Hippocratic approach began, which had not considered infection to catalyse disease or its rapid transmission.

Attention moved to reduce contact with infectious agents, and some discoveries linked pandemics to germ theory. Europe thought epidemics were linked to miasma theory, where environmental factors such as polluted water and poor hygiene were causative agents. Louis Pasteur's discoveries supported the germ theory and its use in treatment.

Medicine understood that environmental factors and hereditary influences would influence how a disease progressed or if a person would become infected. Germ theory gave the cause of infectious diseases. More up-to-date research centres came about early in the 20th century, with new treatments such as antibiotic production. Further progress in chemistry, genetic study, and medical radiography further shaped the medical model we have today.

## The Medical Model

In his book Power Healing, Dr Leo Galland explains that conventional medicine uses the biomedical model. Steps towards diagnosis include the symptoms reported by the patient, previous medical history, and examination. This aims to result in a differential diagnosis of the illness. If more than one condition is possible, more investigations may help, aiming to reduce the risk of missing life-threatening situations, and help to arrive at the correct diagnosis and treatment.

Tests may rule out specific concerns, and referral to a specialist could be the next step. Dr Galland explains the downside of this approach is that more emphasis is given to diagnostic tests rather than what discussion with the patient can provide. There may be a wide variation in a doctor's assessment of a patient and a patient's experience of illness. Many factors can influence how a patient presents, which, without discussion, aren't considered.

The functional medicine approach is more person-centred, considering contributing factors such as life history, and triggers such as trauma, microbes, allergens, toxins, and more. Childhood, illness, all the background stories to this life and what shaped it, may be relevant. Patient enquiry helps uncover and shed light on the individual characteristics of each person. And the unique tapestry woven into the life presented may help uncover circumstances culminating in where illness has arrived.

I read a great deal and joined summits looking for help in the days before I found ReCODE. Precision medicine is seen by many as the way forward, and it is strides ahead in certain areas. It makes interesting reading for anyone wanting to learn more. Each patient is unique, so people may present with the same disease picture but treatment may differ, because predisposing factors might differ. No one size fits all; no standard prescription.

## The Role we Have

President Truman made good use of the phrase "THE BUCK STOPS HERE". And he displayed it on his desk, highlighting he was responsible for any decisions made. This journey led me to consider whether we take enough responsibility for our own health. Dr Sherry A. Rogers writes that we should reach a ripe old age and die in our sleep, yet we accept we will degenerate as we age. It comes with the territory, no questions asked.

The conventional medical model seems to have induced a mindset where we hand ourselves over, expecting the doctor to fix our complaint. Of course, medication will be the only answer at times, but we do not consider looking for an alternative when one might exist. Nor do we question the limitations within the medical model, but it's clear that mainstream medicine is not helping us all.

There's also the attitude that the doctor is always right when, in fact, that may not be the case. A friend I hadn't seen in some time expressed shock at my experience trying to get help with cognitive decline. She was glad I'd persisted, but acknowledged she would have accepted what the doctor told her. I might have, too, if I hadn't witnessed dementia in my family, and I have no doubt I would have ended up in care.

We may believe illness to be unavoidable if it runs in the family – but that isn't a foregone conclusion. If you put people with similar genetics on the same diet, expose them to toxins and similar environmental circumstances, voila! There's a good chance they will develop similar problems and may get the same disease process as their overexposed systems struggle. The website https://www.houstonmethodist.org/ explains this better, as some disease can be inherited; search for inherited diseases on their website.

We should ask: why me? Why did this illness happen to me? We should work with our care provider instead of expecting the doctor to fix everything. The conventional medical model almost encourages us to leave the responsibility with the practitioner and not look for another solution, perhaps believing there isn't one.

I now have a better understanding of why Dad's dementia symptoms were so severe and why SSRI antidepressants didn't help my brother. Recovering from an overload of toxins was a struggle before getting guidance from functional clinicians. It's a struggle we can avoid if we get access to wider health education. Minimal drug use during the Black Death pandemic highlighted the need for more. But now pharmaceutical treatments have become a business in their own right.

This is not to downplay the many significant advances in medicine which allopathy has achieved, and I am personally grateful to the skilled surgeons whose help I've needed. But treatment isn't successful for every cancer. There is currently no medication on the market that can stop the progression of Alzheimer's disease. Yet we can do much to support our wellbeing when given the right advice.

I didn't know this information before, and perhaps cared little, but that changed with an experience of cognitive decline and the hard-hitting reality of no available medical help. Improvement is possible in some conditions if you know what medical approach to seek.

The advances in mainstream medicine over the years may have led us to think of functional medicine as a method from bygone days. But both medical approaches have much to offer. We do not have to choose one approach over the other, but it's time for easier patient access to the best of both systems of medicine. Functional medicine comes at a cost, though, and we may not be prepared for that. It is also rarely covered by health insurance. It's up to the individual patient, if they have health insurance, to see if it will cover the tests needed.

In the United Kingdom, the National Health Service does not take care of Alzheimer's patients once their health declines. Care is in the private care home environment, which has to be paid for. So, the decision may be having to choose whether to invest in yourself now, or invest in care if that is the outcome. I never considered I would need help to ward off dementia, and I never thought the system of medicine in which I nursed could not help me, as many others have experienced.

Our outlook has a significant role in managing our health. Knowledge is power, as the saying goes, and it's time to get better informed. Especially for those of us who have an illness with which mainstream medicine can offer little or no help. I want my family to have knowledge of prevention or hope of improvement if they're already on the way to health issues.

# Chapter 19

# A Patient's Perspective

The years when I struggled before finding ReCODE were chaotic and exhausting, and hope faded. Healing is often non-linear, and misunderstanding and setbacks can leave us questioning if we've made the right choice.

Uncovering the root cause of my symptoms brought understanding of why I went through all I did. Knowing why I developed cognitive symptoms makes a world of a difference. The ReCODE protocol and everything I've learned over these years has renewed hope.

Change isn't easy. A few times on this journey I've caught my breath at the thought of the changes to be made, but the outcome was worth it. More so having witnessed the depth of destruction Alzheimer's can bring in my own family. On telling my family I carried the APoE4 gene and had been having symptoms, I told them to get back to me if they had any questions. My son Adam phrased it well. On checking he understood the news I'd shared he asked, "Am I right in saying you've had this, but if you stick to the rules you'll be fine?" I couldn't have said it better myself, and let's replace rules with lifestyle changes.

If management of your health problems is not bringing improvement and you want more, you have to start somewhere. There are pros and cons to doing what you can on your own, so guidance from a practitioner can be valuable. I became quite unwell trying to detox when I couldn't find help, but I now know that detox pathways need to be working at their best beforehand, which makes sense. Cost can be a concern, but there are several ways to help yourself, and advice can be sought when the time is right.

When symptoms returned, I got up earlier so I could read books that helped me. This was only a few months before I found Dr Bredesen's work, and reading continues to support my health in ways that resonate with me. Second-hand books are often available through Amazon.

Access to free information is available on some practitioner websites, and helpful podcasts and short courses are also available. There are webinars and membership websites you can join on your healing journey, as well as the many books and materials online which can point you in the right direction. Gains can be achieved and later, if finances allow, guidance sought to ensure things are progressing correctly. Lists of such websites can be found in the Appendix.

I read an article in a newspaper once which highlighted that conventional doctors frown upon patients searching on Google. In all honesty, I would have been in care long ago if I hadn't searched online. However, this book would not be a fair representation of the difficulties that may be encountered if I wasn't completely honest. I've expressed my gratitude to the conventional doctors who have helped me while acknowledging some have not, and sadly the functional route has not been without problems.

When I started on this journey in 2013 there was no help for cognitive decline within functional medicine or alternative therapies in the UK. I corresponded with a number of therapists when I thought it was heavy metal toxicity who were honest enough to explain they no longer did chelation. I am also truly grateful to any of the practitioners who have helped me in any way to get back en route to health. However, I have on four occasions found myself left in the lurch, up the creek without a paddle, abandoned, dumped... take your pick. This has happened with three different functional/alternative therapist clinics and one holistic dentist.

I don't know if the "no response" approach is particular to Scotland but its off-putting if having to consider the functional approach.

## Avoiding Such Pitfalls

Diet is one of the main things affecting us, and getting off the processed diet alone will be a significant steppingstone to well-being. Dr Cari Schaeffer's book The Food Solution explains what we should not be eating and gives different plans for transitioning off processed food at your own pace. The aforementioned websites can provide guidance. Once again knowledge is power. The more informed you are the more questions you can ask that are relevant to any health issues you are dealing with. Some websites can give access to practitioners they have trained, for example the websites of Dr. Nirala Jacobi and Dr Terry Wahls (please see appendix B).

Read about any therapist you may be considering. What are they offering? What training have they completed? Do they have any area of expertise? If clarity calls are offered, take the benefit of them to get any questions you may have answered.

If you want to prevent cognitive decline, Dr Bredesens's book The End of Alzheimer's PROGRAMME may be all you need. Bear in mind I found it an overwhelming read, but as individuals we do not have all predisposing factors and so not all the information will apply to you.

Should you need ReCODE, let me start by saying I will be eternally grateful Dr Bredesen's initial training was put out into the world. But this has been an expensive journey for me for various reasons.

Firstly the toxic subtype is the most difficult to treat, and you have to go slow. The situation in my gut took two years to manifest as symptoms that suggested for sure something needed attention. This undoubtedly stood in my way, indicated inflammation, and clouded the picture for practitioners. I also believed I had difficulty detoxing, but I was attending the clinic for over a year before it became clear that I did. Again, this would have been standing in my way of moving forward.

Much can be gained from the book for anyone needing ReCODE but more help is in your best interest as you want to discover the "why" and manage it. You can assess your cognitive health for free through the Apollo Health website. The website gives the option of a subscription membership for both prevention and ReCODE, or you can search for a practitioner yourself.

I have not had a subscription membership, because initially it was felt it wasn't needed as I did a lot to help myself. The health coach explained the benefits of a membership but, on the basis of what I'd already spent, I decided not to take it so that I could meet the cost of further tests.

The benefits from a subscription membership for ReCODE include a personalised generated report, as your practitioner will input your test results. Such results will still be discussed with you if you don't have a membership, just in a different format. There is also access to meetings and other resources. Most importantly, should your case become difficult to understand, Dr Bredesen can then work with your practitioner to offer advice, and so that may be your preference.

Telemedicine allows easy access to practitioners no matter their location. If searching for your own practitioner or coach through the website search facility, you'll then get the practitioner's details through Apollo Health. Visit practitioner websites and see what is offered. Get a clarity call to get your questions answered. Once you discover your "why"it may be beneficial to get input from a therapist who specialises in that area. If you need ReCODE, you will be investing in yourself, so you want to invest wisely.

I needed a practitioner for blood tests and advice on supplements. And I decided to have a health coach, as it was hard work doing all the research I previously did on my own. It was good to have the insight of someone trained in the protocol who could assist me in the best way to do it. But you don't have to have a practitioner and coach at the same time, if choosing both. There will be time between your initial screening results and reviewing how you're doing on the protocol. You may decide to see a health coach during that period, or later if that suits better. But getting onto the protocol is going to help with some things highlighted in the screening, and that's where a ReCODE 2 .0 Health Coach is a great benefit.

# Chapter 20

# Revisiting the Brain Scan

I understand that environmental illness is not the area of expertise within conventional medicine, and you can't treat what you don't know. But sometimes when a conventional practitioner doesn't know, the patient is dismissed and might not realise there is another way.

Let me go back to my brain scan report. Cerebral small vessel disease (SVD) relates to aberrations in the brain's small blood vessels, and it is a very common problem – more so in older adults. It's been linked to the white matter issues and vascular ischaemia, as reported on my brain scan. However, due to its common occurrence, it would appear it doesn't perhaps get the recognition it deserves from our primary healthcare services. And that's certainly a problem for anyone wanting early detection of possible dementia symptoms.

When I went for advice on the brain scan report, I was told by a doctor that she didn't know what it meant for me, as she wasn't a neurologist. Okay, fair point. But she said a scan of her brain would probably show the same damage. So its common occurrence would appear to downplay what it might be a precursor of. And there are concerning problems linked to SVD when it's moderate or severe, which the Better Health While Aging website mentions as:

- Difficulties with balance and walking. (I leaned over to the one side when walking when balance episodes occurred, with the exception of the day when I needed the support of my kitchen table. Vertigo was too intense that day to even consider trying to walk.)
- Cognitive impairment.
- An increase in the risk of stroke.
- It can indicate vascular dementia or the possibility of developing it.
- Research has concluded it is linked to an increased risk or increased severity of Alzheimer's disease and other dementias.

My family history, and the fact that I knew I shared symptoms with my relatives, was why I had been seeking help in primary care since 2012-2013. The scan results indicate why I was having the symptoms I experienced. I can excuse the fact that in 2013 my symptoms weren't recognised, since I learned that's not unusual with the toxic subtype of Alzheimer's. But am I wrong in thinking that the brain scan should have led to me being taken more seriously?

Let me touch on increased severity of Alzheimer disease, as witnessed with my dad's decline. Within a short period of time following diagnosis, my dad's language was garbled. As expected, at times he didn't recognise family members, and he developed an obsession with money, so we had to get him a purse and small chain so it could be attached to his trousers to ease this anxiety for him. These things were manageable.

The more heartbreaking developments saw him weep due to the way he was feeling. He lost the ability to read – something he enjoyed daily. He needed help with personal care and became doubly incontinent. He lost stones in weight, which a psychiatrist explained to me was due to the disease having spread to the metabolic regions of his brain. And he went on to need assistance with feeding.

He became ataxic, and it was actually falling that led to his admission to hospital. That's why his remaining years were spent in a recliner chair for his own safety. Nearer the end of his life, he had difficulty swallowing without choking. Food was pureed, and fluids were thickened with a product called Thick and Easy, which I'd personally rather be dehydrated than have to take. I'm sharing this because there is no guarantee that a person will get 'a little bit' of dementia.

The fact is that same brain scan has now been filed as normal with my doctor's surgery, so I can only be truly grateful I found ReCODE before it was too late for me to return from the cognitive issues. Sadly, this lack of detection isn't uncommon for dementia sufferers. For me, the alarming thing is that some people with a family history seem to see it coming, like myself, while doctors don't – perhaps a reflection that mainstream medicine can currently offer no help.

I've read of others who, on voicing their concerns, received glib comments from the doctor they were looking to for advice. And it's not just in the UK. Francis C. McNear, in his book Defeating Dementia, disclosed information from the Alzheimer Association in America that the amount of people or their carers who actually got a diagnosis of Alzheimer's dementia was 45%.

On the one hand, I'll admit I'm glad the doctor did not refer me to the memory clinic. Had I attended for assessment, the cognitive deficits I initially showed, and other results, could have led to the suggestion that dementia might be approaching and I could have lost hope. However, it would have been good to have access to some of the investigations, such as a brain scan when needed, to confirm my experience.

I also like the fact that the ReCODE protocol has no side effects to be concerned about, while drugs do. And I'm not going to say I would never consider medication if I arrived at a diagnosis of Alzheimer's, but that choice would be dependent on whether the medication worked, which it didn't for my relatives. For now, though, I don't need medication for Alzheimer's disease, and I don't because I found ReCODE.

I've pondered if Alzheimer's disease could be considered the Black Death of our time, in as much as it clearly highlights that more is needed than the medical care we have access to can offer. Early detection is helpful for those who want an alternative approach to managing cognitive decline.

Neither am I playing down how hard making changes is. But if things don't change, our younger generation has little to look forward to.

# Chapter 21

# Our Children

Age-wise, my dad presented with dementia a decade earlier than his mother did. And I presented with cognitive issues a decade earlier than him. Besides how our current lifestyle affects our health, we should consider the future of our children, as they are becoming unwell to a greater degree. Dr Sherry Rodgers states that childhood cancers are higher than before and are the principal cause of death through illness in the 1-to-15-year age group.

Girls are experiencing puberty at an earlier age, along with the physical changes and mood swings. There are more cases of undescended testicles in boys, hypospadias, and testicular cancer. Endocrine disruptors from environmental toxins are contributing to this in our young, and such toxins may also contribute to fertility issues, problems with menstruation, and cysts. The brain is affected, too, leading to behavioural and learning difficulties, and the resulting weakened immunity contributes to allergies and infections.

Dr Natasha Campbell-McBride is also a mum, who helped her child recover from autism. She devoted her work to assisting families facing similar issues and noticed an increase in other conditions in children. These include ADHD, ADD, behavioural and learning difficulties, dyslexia, asthma, dyspraxia, allergies, and eczema. Some children experiencing these conditions later received a diagnosis of depression, bipolar disorder, schizophrenia, or other psychological and psychiatric issues.

A significant underlying factor to these conditions was the child's digestive health, as it's linked to their mental development. Dr Campbell-McBride named the disorder gut and psychology syndrome, or Gap syndrome, to describe where gut health can lead to the above conditions.

Dr Cate Shanahan explains that she has seen physiological deterioration in our young because of dietary changes over generations; the elders in a family would be healthier than the younger members of the family. She noted that the earlier the processed diet was eaten, the greater the deterioration, due to a diet that's both nutrient deficient and contains chemicals absent in the food of our ancestors.

We haven't questioned such effects on our young, perhaps because mainstream medicine doesn't make that causal link, so we accept such changes as normal. Asthma and ear infections are a few of the ones we're more acquainted with, to serious issues such as a hole in the heart or some other surgery that's needed in childhood. While medication may manage the symptoms, much of this inheritance is the lack of nutritional value in the processed diet.

We need to become more aware, as children don't deserve the inheritance our current way of living passes onto them. A newborn's microbiome is influenced by both parents and continues to develop after the birth. But if the mum and dad's gut flora is out of sync, baby starts life with a compromised microbiome. And toxins can be passed to baby through breastfeeding.

It's our responsibility to educate ourselves and improve our health to benefit the children we bring into this world. We have a significant role to play in making our children's future a healthy one. The processed diet, prescription medication, toxins, and lack of care for the microbiome, aren't only leading us down the path of degenerative disease. The mental and physical health of our young is also being affected.

## Autism

Autism is on the rise, and we should be asking why. It's unknown if genetics has a role, but genetics alone does not explain the increase in the incidence.

We're aware of the furore questioning a link between vaccination and autism, and the MMR vaccine is not the only vaccine that's been considered a potential link. Besides Dr Andrew Wakefield's research linking inflammatory bowel with autism, other research has supported his findings. For many children, vaccination won't be a trigger, but for some, it might be the ultimate thing that tips the child onto the autistic spectrum.

Dr Campbell-McBride feels it's not as straightforward to link vaccination to autism, and that the bigger picture has to be considered. Many of the illnesses presenting in our young share a weakened immune system. A weak immune system will not accept vaccination as well as an immune system that functions more effectively, and vaccine administration is aimed at a healthy immune system.

She states that any weakened immune system will lead to illness, even in the absence of vaccination. She has witnessed this in her practice with children who have not been vaccinated but develop autism or other Gap conditions. Our modern lifestyle is at the root of weakened immunity in our young.

I read of two five-year-olds who recovered from autism when treated as coeliac disease. One with the treatment itself; the other got a resolution of gut issues, after which his autism symptoms ceased. The medics from the University of Atlanta advised that screening for coeliac disease and nutritional deficiency could be helpful for those with neurological conditions, including autistic spectrum disorder.

Various approaches have helped some children recover, and often a combination of methods is needed. Detox homeopathy has been helpful for some children on the autistic spectrum. Julie Matthews is a Nutritional Consultant and researcher. Back in 2001, she found that nutrition could positively affect autism. She investigated further and published an award-winning book, Nourishing Hope for Autism.

She later learned that diet could be helpful for most chronic illnesses and uses nutrition to help teens and adults, too. There may be various factors contributing to autism, and everyone is individual so may have different contributors. But digestive health and diet have a central role in improvement. As well as autism, Julie Matthews' work treats many of the conditions presenting in our young today.

It's another health journey for parents that requires much effort, and one that often takes place over a long period. However, referring to the effort recovery may take, Dr Campbell-McBride said, "...but being a parent of a recovered child myself, I can tell you it's one of the most rewarding experiences on earth."

## Vaccination

It was by the late 1940s that vaccination as a method of disease control was available on a large-scale. Recommended routine vaccination for pertussis, diphtheria, and tetanus were combined in 1948. And the list of vaccines has increased over the years. The current UK Immunisation Schedule includes a 6-in-1 vaccine from eight weeks old, which is repeated at 12 and 16 weeks, in addition to other vaccines that are given alongside it. That's a lot for an infant gut to handle.

I thought the movie Vaxxed must be anti-vaccination, however, the website publicises that a 2004 study withheld data suggesting a link between the MMR vaccine and autism. And it is not asking for vaccine removal, but for the availability of separate vaccines.

None of us wants to go back to pre-vaccination times when many died. However, the subject deserves more consideration when our children's health is not at its best. Dr Campbell-McBride feels medicine should give more attention to assessing a child's suitability for vaccination rather than immunising all children before a certain age. She advises that assessment should be based on the child's level of immunity, gut health, and parental health. Thereafter, knowledge gained would show if it's safe for vaccination to go ahead as planned, or if there should be a delay, or even omission.

## Chapter 22

# The Legend of the Rainbow Warrior

I t's clear that our so-called modern lifestyle is overexposing us to toxins and a less nutritious diet of processed food, and for some of us it's hazardous to health.

To my embarrassment, before this wake-up call I took nothing to do with current affairs, politics, environmental issues, or any causes. It could have been laziness, but underlying it all, I guess I felt such things didn't affect me, so I felt no responsibility to keep up-to-date or take an interest. I have, however, always felt passionate about what happens to our children, and I firmly believe we have a responsibility to look after them if we bring them into this world.

This journey has shown me how little attention I paid to the harm we do to our environment and to our bodies by our modern way of life. I've explained the detrimental effects of the processed diet and the toxins we're surrounded by: a slow decline if we're lucky; degenerative disease if we're not.

Another reason I was perhaps not proactive on various issues is that I tend to be an introvert, yet the youth of today are speaking out for climate change. Their example makes me wonder if I can use my introversion as an excuse to do nothing. The changes I've had to make because of mycotoxin illness has helped my home environment and my health. That might be all I can do, but I intend to stay informed now, and if I can help contribute to a better tomorrow in some way, I will. The outcome for future generations is up to us.

The rainbow is a revered symbol among Native American traditions. To the Navajo, it is the path of the holy spirits. The Cherokee describes it as the "hem of the sun's coat". It's also understood as a sign of unity among people.

Sun Bear, an Ojibwe teacher and author, tells of prophecies relating that people of all races will come back as the Rainbow Warriors to aid the restoration of Mother Earth. Many versions of the rainbow prophecy exist, but the consistent message is the need for peace, healing, and unity.

Many believe that the devastation to the earth described in the prophesies is happening in our time. Pollution is affecting sea life. The bee population has declined. Butterflies and bugs are experiencing a cataclysmic decrease, and other animals and plants are dying because of changes in their environment. An account of the legend from the Cree tradition explains that the Warriors of the Rainbow would help people understand what to do to help them live in harmony, bringing healing to Mother Earth. They will need to stand firm, as there will be opposition, but change is the only way back.

Delwin Fiddler Jr. conveys in his blog that we are the change-makers, the Rainbow Warriors of the prophecies. It's how we act now that allows the generations that follow to flourish. The long-lasting impact of the damage done will only be reversed by taking action.

It's our children's birthright to be born into a world that will not harm them. We must be mindful of how our choices affect the world they inherit. It's time to do what we can to heal ourselves. It's time to do what we can to revere Mother Earth. We have the opportunity to act and to awaken the Rainbow Warrior within.

# End Notes

All information correct at the time of publishing.

### Chapter 3 - My Plight Begins

- Amalgam Illness diagnosis and treatment by Andrew Hall Cutler. ISBN 0-9676168-0-8
- https://quackwatch.org/chelation/reports/provoked/

### Chapter 5 - Take Two

- https://pubmed.ncbi.nlm.nih.gov/31876406/
- https://pubmed.ncbi.nlm.nih.gov/34841505/#:
  ~:text=Small%20intestinal%20bacterial%20overgrowt
  h%20(SIBOand%20SIBO%20has%20been%20establis
  hed

### Chapter 7 - The Research

- The End of Alzheimers by Dr Dale Bredesen.
  ISBN 978-1-78504-122-8
- 'Regain Your Brain Summit' – Interview with Peggy Sarlin and Dr Dale Bredesen.
- https://microbeminded.com/2017/12/18/interview-with-robert-moir-infection-in-alzheimers-brain-microbiome/
- https://www.verywellhealth.com/amyloid-cascade-hypothesis-of-alzheimers-disease-98791

## Chapter 8 - My Diagnosis

- The End of Alzheimers by Dr Dale Bredesen.
  ISBN 978-1-78504-122-8
- https://pubmed.ncbi.nlm.nih.gov/2618578/
- https://www.hindawi.com/journals/jar/2011/617927

## Chapter 9 - My Other Contributors

- https://www.webmd.com/a-to-z-guides/what-is-physiology
- https://pubmed.ncbi.nlm.nih.gov/25402818/
  This is a link to Dr. Leo Galland's article 'The Gut Microbiome and the Brain'.
- Article by Angelucci F, Cechova K, Amlerova J, Hort. 'Antibiotics, Gut Microbiota and Alzheimer Disease'.
- https://gutgeek.com/
- https://selfhacked.com/blog/lipopolysaccharides/
- https://justinhealth.com/leaky-gut-syndrome/
- https://qbi.uq.edu.au/brain/brain-anatomy/what-blood-brain-barrier
- The Food Solution by Dr Cari Schaeffer.
  ISBN 9781518824418
- https://nyulangone.org/conditions/celiac-disease-gluten-sensitivity-in-adults/diagnosis
- https://www.mindbodygreen.com/articles/what-is-gliadin
- https://www.kalishinstitute.com/blog/the-methodology-of-gluten
- Grain Brain by Dr David Perlmutter.
  ISBN 978-1-473-69558-0.
- https://www.tuw.edu/health/how-stress-affects-the-brain/
- https://www.mayoclinic.org/healthy-lifestyle/stress-

management/in-depth/stress/art-20046037

## Chapter 11 - Dietary Revelations

- https://cks.nice.org.uk/topics/rheumatoid-arthritis/
  diagnosis/investigations-for-suspected-ra/
- https://www.ncbi.nlm.nih.gov/pmc/articles/
  PMC3641836/
  This article describes psychiatric and neurological
  symptoms in relation to gluten sensitivity and the
  difference between gluten sensitivity and coeliac
  disease.
- https://glutenfreeworks.com/blog/2017/07/15/
  celiac-rage-and-nutritional-deficiencies/
  Link to article on how gluten and nutrient deficiencies
  may affect us.
- https://www.kalishinstitute.com/blog/the-
  methodology-of-gluten

## Chapter 12 - More Changes Needed

- http://journeytoforever.org/text_price.html
  Information on Dr Weston Price.
- Nourishing Diets by Sally Fallon Morell.
  ISBN 978-1-5387-1168-2
- Deep Nutrition by Catherine Shanahan M.D.
  ISBN 978-1-250-11384-9
- The Wahls Protocol by Terry Wahls M.D.
  ISBN 978-1-58333-554-3
- Gut and Psychology Syndrome by Dr. Natasha
  Campbell-McBride M.D. ISBN 0-9548520-2-8
- Dirty Genes by Dr. Ben Lynch.
  ISBN 978-0-06269815-5

- Chris Beat Cancer By Chris Wark.
  ISBN 978-1-78817-529-6

## Chapter 13 - Supported by Spirit

- https://www.jacquelynelane.com/
- http://www.vkmaheshwari.com/WP/
- http://www.differencebetween.net/miscellaneous/
  culture-miscellaneous/differences-between-nymphs-
  and-fairies/
- https://en.wikipedia.org/wiki/Deva_(New_Age)
- https://eskildtjalve.dk/
- https://health.clevelandclinic.org/cayenne-pepper-
  benefits/
- https://www.hyperbiotics.com/blogs/recent-articles/
  the-fascinating-truth-behind-tomatoes-and-gut-health
- https://food.ndtv.com/food-drinks/9-incredible-
  benefits-of-basil-leaves-you-may-not-have-known-
  1834742

## Chapter 15 - A New Way of Being

- https://www.safecosmetics.org/chemicals/titanium-
  dioxide/

## Chapter 16 - Dietary Confusion

- https://www.diabetes.co.uk/in-depth/every-last-shred-
  evidence-low-fat-dietary-guidelines-never-introduced/
- The Fatburn Fix by Catherine Shanahan M.D.
  ISBN 978-1-250-11449-5
- The Wahls Protocol by Terry Wahls M.D.
  ISBN 978-1-58333-554-3
- Deep Nutrition by Catherine Shanahan M.D.

ISBN 978-1-250-11384-9

- The Food Solution by Dr Cari Schaeffer.
  ISBN 9781518824418
- Dirty Genes by Dr. Ben Lynch.
  ISBN 978-0=06269815-5
- https://www.cdc.gov/genomics/disease/epigenetics.
  htm#~:text=Epigenetics%20is%20the%20study%20of,
  body%20reads%20a%20DNA%20sequence

## Chapter 17 - We Live in a Toxic World

- Detoxify or Die by Sherry A Rogers M.D.
  ISBN 1-887202-04-8
- https://www.cambridge.org/core/journals/the-british-
  journal-of-psychiatry/article/aluminium-and-fluoride-
  in-drinking-water-in-relation-to-later-dementia-risk/
  14AF4F22AC68C9D6F34F9EC91BE37B6D
  Search function on website may need to be used for
  article to display.
- https://www.safecosmetics.org/
- https://ynatural.com.au/ingredients-to-avoid/
  ingredient-avoid-disodium-edta/
- https://www.annmariegianni.com/ingredient-watch-
  list-tetrasodium-edta-the-preservative-made-from-
  formaldehyde/
- https://metro.co.uk/2020/11/20/drinking-coffee-
  from-disposable-cups-could-be-seriously-bad-for-you-
  13626234/8-
- https://pubmed.ncbi.nlm.nih.gov/12396676/
- https://www.thespinalcentre.com.au/is-aluminium-
  really-safe/

- https://www.ncbi.nlm.nih.gov/pmc/articles/
  PMC3056430/
  A link between Aluminum and the Pathogenesis of
  Alzheimer's Disease: 'The Integration of the
  Aluminum and Amyloid Cascade Hypotheses'.

## Chapter 18 - The Changing Face of Medicine

- https://www.britannica.com/science/history-of-
  medicine#ref35642
- https://www.greeka.com/greece-history/famous-
  people/hippocrates/
- https://www.livescience.com/62515-hippocrates.html
- https://study.com/academy/lesson/the-four-humors-
  lesson-quiz.html
- Thesis by Vanneste, Sarah Frances, 'The Black Death
  And The Future Of Medicine' (2010)
- https://en.wikipedia.org/wiki/History_of_medicine
- Power Healing by Leo Galland M.D.
  ISBN 978-0-375-75139-4
- https://en.wikipedia.org/wiki/Buck_
  passing#References

## Chapter 20 - Revisiting the Brain Scan

- https://betterhealthwhileaging.net/cerebral-small-
  vessel-disease/

## Chapter 21 - Our Children

- Detoxify or Die by Sherry A Rogers M.D.
  ISBN 1-887202-04-8
- Gut and Psychology Syndrome. ISBN 0-9548520-2-8
- https://glutenfreeworks.com/blog/2021/07/14/can-

celiac-disease-be-mistaken-as-autism-a-boy-whose-autism-was-cured/

- https://nourishinghope.com/
- https://www.chop.edu/centers-programs/vaccine-education-center/vaccine-history/developments-by-year
- https://vk.ovg.ox.ac.uk/uk-schedule
- https://vaxxedthemovie.com/
- Deep Nutrition by Catherine Shanahan M.D. ISBN 978-1-250-11384-9

## Chapter 22 - The Legend of the Rainbow Warrior

- https://en.wikipedia.org/wiki/Rainbows_in_mythology
- https://theearthstoriescollection.org/en/the-legend-of-the-rainbow-warriors/
- https://blog.nativehope.org/the-rainbow-warrior

# Appendix A

## Helpful Books

- The End of Alzheimer's by Dr Dale Bredesen.
  ISBN 978-1-78504-122-8
  Introduction to ReCODE, and the science behind the
  ReCODE protocol.
- The End of Alzheimer's Programme by Dr Dale
  Bredesen. ISBN 978-1-78504-227-0
  A resource of new information, how to use the
  concepts to improve your cognition and more.
- Detoxify or Die by Sherry A Rogers M.D.
  ISBN 1-887202-04-8
  Dr Rogers' book highlights the extent to which toxin
  exposure is affecting us.
- Living a Life Less Toxic by Faith Canter.
  ISBN 978-0-9957047-4-9
- Dirty Genes by Dr. Ben Lynch.
  ISBN 978-0-06-269815-5
  Dr Lynch advises on how to clean up our genes.
- Toxic Heal Your Body by Neil Nathan M.D.
  ISBN 978-1-628603-11-8
  Useful information on difficult to treat conditions and
  ways to help turn that around.
- Clean & Green by Nancy Birtwhistle.
  ISBN-13: 978-1529049725 Eco-friendly cleaning.

- At Home With Aromatherapy by Faye Willmott.
  ISBN 978-1-7396283-0-7
  A resource for using aromatherapy at home.

## Books That Helped me with Dietary Choices

One caution I must add is that many books will advise wholegrain brown rice. As I was dealing with toxins, white rice is best, as arsenic can be in the outer layers of brown rice.

- Gut and Psychology Syndrome by Dr. Natasha Campbell-McBride M.D. ISBN 0-9548520-2-8
- The Wahls Protocol by Terry Wahls M.D.
  ISBN 978-1-58333-554-3
- The Food Solution by Dr Cari Schaeffer.
  ISBN 9781518824418
  Helpful guidance on moving away from processed food. Dr Cari also gives plans to help you start.
- Deep Nutrition by Catherine Shanahan M.D.
  ISBN 978-1-250-11384-9
- The Fatburn Fix by Catherine Shanahan M.D.
  ISBN 978-1-250-11449-5
- Nourishing Traditions by Sally Fallon.
  ISBN 0-96708973-5
- THE WHOLESOME yum EASY KETO COOKBOOK by Maya Krampf.
  ISBN 978-1-9848-2662-6
- Quick & easy KETOGENIC COOKING by Maria Emmerich. ISBN 978-1-628601-00-8

# Appendix B

## Useful Websites

- https://www.apollohealthco.com/
  Access to a free cognitive assessment. You can search
  for practitioners to work alone or subscription
  memberships are available to PreCODE for
  prevention of cognitive decline or ReCODE for
  people needing the protocol.
- https://www.thecognitivehealthcoach.co.uk/
- https://www.gapsdiet.com/
- https://breakingtheviciouscycle.info/
  The website for the specific carbohydrate diet.
- https://drcate.com/
  Dr. Cate Shanahan's website gives information on her
  books. There are many articles providing information
  and free resources.
- https://terrywahls.com/
  Dr Wahls' website. A resource for managing Multiple
  Sclerosis and autoimmune conditions.
- https://drjessmd.com/about/
  A membership functional medicine website called
  Wellness Plus. It has much useful information.
  However, Fullscript does not ship supplements
  internationally. Working with a practitioner may be
  helpful for that. You can sign up to the mailing list, or
  follow on social media to get an insight into what's
  available to help decide if Wellness Plus is valuable to
  you.
- https://www.drterrawinston.com/
  A functional medicine website with an informative

blog and access to more.

You can sign up to the mailing list, or follow on social media to get an insight into what's available.

- https:/www.thesibodoctor.com//
  Dr. Nirala Jacobi's website. Patient course and podcast available.
- https://www.siboinfo.com/
  Informative website with access to many resources.
- https://goodbyeleakygut.com/
  Resources for leaky gut.
- https://www.westonaprice.org/#gsc.tab=0
  The Weston Price Foundation
- https://offallygoodcooking.com/
  A resource for learning how to cook offal.
- https://glutenfreeworks.com/
- https://www.luvele.co.uk/
  Appliances and recipes to support a healthy lifestyle.
- https://www.pan-uk.org/
  For information of the dirty dozen vegetable and fruit list.
- https://www.ewg.org/foodnews/dirty-dozen.php
  Environmental Working Group – updated information on dirty dozen list.
- https://thegoodlifedesigns.com/non-toxic-kitchenware-guide/
  A guide to help reduce toxins in the kitchen.
- https://www.safecosmetics.org/chemicals/
  Chemicals of concern we should be avoiding.
- https://www.cheonline.co.uk/the-home-prescriber-course
  Free online course for using homeopathy at home.

# Help For Parents

- https://nourishinghope.com/
  A nutritional approach for autism and ADHD.
- http://pecanbread.com/
  This website offers advice for children on the specific carbohydrate diet for gut issues and/or autism. Julie Matthews has found some autistic children on the specific carbohydrate diet still need some other dietary tweaks.
- https://nourishingourchildren.org/
  An educational resource from the Weston Price Foundation.
- https://rita-kara-robinson.com/
  Detox Homeopathy. Vaccine injury specialist for autism, Gardasil, and general health issues.

# Some of the Websites I Use

- https://eversfieldorganic.co.uk/
  Rewards scheme available.
- https://www.coombefarmorganic.co.uk/
  Rewards scheme available.
- https://www.lovingfoods.co.uk/
  Fermented food and drinks.
- https://nutspick.co.uk/
- https://frejafoods.com/
  While I make bone broth, it's been handy having this broth to hand. Good for a keto diet, too.
- https://www.buywholefoodsonline.co.uk/
- https://lizza.net/
  I make keto rolls and freeze them, but when life takes over I use Lizza's keto bread range and freeze in slices.

- https://www.champohaircare.com/
- https://mgnaturals.com/
  Titanium-free makeup. Etsy store available for UK and EU orders.
- https://friendlysoap.co.uk/
- https://lailalondon.com/
  Facial oils.
- https://www.biggreensmile.com/
- https://www.neovite.com/
  Best value-for-money colostrum.
- https://skyecandles.co.uk/
  Free shipping in the UK. Rewards scheme available.

# About the Author

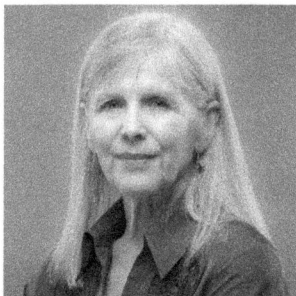

I rene Smith originally trained as a Registered General Nurse and went on to obtain an Orthopaedic Nursing Certificate. She staffed in Orthopaedics and later Care of the Elderly over a twenty five year period. She established a Complimentary Therapy Practice in 2006 which remained open till Covid19 led her to decide to move to working from home.

Shamanic practice gives her a way of connecting to the unseen help she has often been aware of and she has trained in many healing modalities.

At the time of writing Irene's website is irenesmith.uk. Email ismith.uk@mail.com. Current facebook page is https://www.facebook.com/ccismith and instagram page https://www.instagram.com/irenesmith.uk/

www.ingramcontent.com/pod-product-compliance
Lightning Source LLC
Chambersburg PA
CBHW031155020426
42333CB00013B/673